D0412463

NEVER SAY DIET

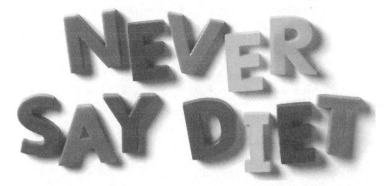

NEVER SAY DIET

Perfect Body · Total Vitality · Complete Well-being

Drew Fobbester

ARCTURUS

About the author

DREW FOBBESTER is a registered nutrition consultant and professional motivator. He is founder and Managing Director of the UK's leading nutrition consultancy, MyNutrition.co.uk, and has executed the UK's largest ever survey relating food intake to well-being. He is a certified fitness instructor and personal trainer as well as a master practitioner and trainer of NLP (the science of human motivation).

He is married to Katie, a registered homoeopath, certified fitness instructor and personal trainer. Together they have run successful private health and training studios both in the UK and on continental Europe.

Drew and Katie live in Surrey with their five children. Drew has spent over twenty years in international corporate management roles. He is no stranger to the demands of modern life – the conflicts and pressures of work, home, relationships, children and family.

Drew has formulated Livetetics from real experience with real people: himself, friends, family and over 50,000 private and corporate clients. Livetetics is born of the results of these experiences.

For my children, Molly, Zoe, Jemma, Kelly and Alex. In the hope that I might continue to help halt at least a portion of the ignorruption in your world.

And for my wife and soul mate, Katie.

Arcturus Publishing Limited
26/27 Bickels Yard
151–153 Bermondsey Street
London SE1 3HA

Published in association with
foulsham
W. Foulsham & Co. Ltd,
The Publishing House, Bennetts Close, Cippenham,
Slough, Berkshire SL1 5AP, England

ISBN 0-572-03131-9

British Library Cataloguing-in-Publication Data: a catalogue record for this book is available from the British Library

This edition printed in 2005

Project editor: Belinda Jones
Book design: Steve West
Cover photography: Will White
Cover design: Peter Ridley and Beatriz Waller

Printed in U.K.

For more information on Livetetics, and Drew Fobbester, go to www.livetetics.com

Livetetics is a registered trademark – Livetetics®

With many thanks for the front cover concept to Charlie Waterhouse and his team at Aqueduct Design and Advertising, 85 Clerkenwell Road, London EC1R 5AR

With thanks to MyNutrition.co.uk for permission to reproduce the charts on pages 144 and 237 – extracts from the 2005 ONUK survey of 37,000 adults

With thanks to Dr Ben Brooksbank for his support and insights in reviewing the manuscript

Contents

FOREWORD

In my experience there are people who live their philosophies and there are people who preach. I have known Drew Fobbester for nearly 10 years. He and his wife Katie are among those people who practise what they believe and the results speak for themselves. They are in great shape and have five fantastic, robustly healthy children who have never had to see a doctor.

I have worked with Drew a great deal over the years and have seen the positive results he achieves with his online consultancy at MyNutrition.co.uk. The results he and his nutrition team achieve with their corporate and personal clients are outstanding. I have worked with Drew and his team with the senior managers of major, blue chip global companies and experienced, first-hand, extraordinary improvements in groups of managers, including increased energy, productivity, ability to deal with stress, weight reduction, lowered cholesterol and freedom from digestive and skin problems, among many others. The sysytem of Livetetics is truly born out of experience and results.

Nutrition, like politics and religion, often generates a very passionate response from people. All three are founded on belief systems that, very often, do not respond well to the suggestion of change. But clearly change is required if we and our children are to live optimally healthy lives in perfect well-being. Livetetics confronts many established views and dogma in nutrition and explains why there can be such confusion and misinformation on what is 'right' versus 'wrong', 'healthy' versus 'unhealthy' or 'balanced' versus 'unbalanced'.

This book raises fundamental issues and should be looked at closely by government officials, legislators, parents, teachers and any nutrition 'expert' who is giving advice to anyone about optimizing their food or nutrient intake. It is imperative that all of these groups start to look deeper into what works rather than what the experts say is 'true'. Drew describes a process of corruption through ignorance as 'ignorruption' – this is a very powerful way of explaining how individuals can be encouraged to believe falsehoods and how science can be manipulated for commercial rather than public interest. Livetetics encourages individuals to look to themselves to find references for the truth.

Livetetics urges us all to try a new way and, only then, to judge the results for ourselves.

Among the many important revelations in Livetetics is the fact that 'all calories are not equal'. Drew makes it clear that the quality of what we eat is much more important than the quantity of what we eat. This has profound implications for the diet and food industry. According to Livetetic principles, the poor quality of the calories that people eat day-to-day is making them incrementally less healthy; and this is just made worse when diet programmes encourage restriction in calorific intake without encouraging fundamental changes in the quality of those calories.

Drew's skill as a motivator of human change comes out in this book. He is a specialist in driving behavioural change by helping people change their beliefs in a positive way. Livetetics will certainly challenge the beliefs of many. The information in this book includes sensible, down-to-earth advice about how to think, how to breathe, how to move, how to drink and how to eat. All of these are critical to our well-being.

Livetetics sets out a new agenda that encourages individuals to take personal responsibility for their health and well-being. But, if we are to do this effectively, we need advice based on results rather than on some fabrication of 'science' or 'common wisdom' that is used to further the interests of global manufacturers. In Livetetics we discover why so much of what we believe to be 'true' can be rather less than helpful. As Drew suggests, there cannot be personal responsibility without impartial information and education – Livetetics sets out to redress the balance. It is based on results and it works. I commend it to you.

Patrick Holford, 2005
Founder of the Institute of Optimum Nutrition
Author of *The Optimum Nutrition Bible*

What is Livetetics?

Your potential is for unlimited well-being. A lean body, perfect skin, abundant energy, total resilience, absolute self-confidence, incredible staying power, extraordinary relationships – total well-being.

This well-being is very easy to obtain. But you have to know where to look for it. We know we could look and feel so much better but how? We know that diets (in the sense of following a commercialized, 'special' diet in order to lose weight) don't work, yet there is always the temptation to try another. We know that some foods are best not eaten yet we continue to eat them. We were never really taught how to think, how to breathe, how to drink, how to move, how to eat – yet these are all fundamental to how and what we are.

Livetetics delivers real strategies for real people. It exposes myths, debunks fads and provides an answer to our health crisis. In the developed world we can expect to die up to 50 years before our time of unnecessary and debilitating degenerative diseases. Heart disease, diabetes, cancer – all virtually non-existent in the natural world – have become the destiny for three-quarters of the civilized world. We are fat, droopy, lethargic, depressed, impotent, infertile, have bad breath and die of totally unnecessary diseases.

Livetetics delivers answers. It combines the brilliant, effective simplicity of the nature doctor with the holistic view of the results-oriented practitioner. It brings in solid experience of twenty-first-century nutrition and merges it with ancient teachings. It shatters the myths of nutrition and disease created by commercial interests that manipulate science, media and government to propagate confusing ideas about what is 'healthy'.

Livetetics is the means by which you can achieve
TOTAL BODY TRANSFORMATION

Livetetics teaches the elusive secrets of clear thinking, positive nutrition and effective lifestyle that guarantee mind-clearing, energy-giving, body-shaping, muscle-toning, strength-building, stress-relieving health and vitality.

Livetetics is a work based on results. There are many people who disagree with the advice that you will find in this book. Many highly educated, very intelligent and well-intentioned people do not accept some of the principles in Livetetics.

Livetetics challenges common beliefs and common wisdom – it has discovered that, when it comes to health and well-being, wisdom is pretty uncommon. When it comes to weight loss it is virtually non-existent. Livetetics challenges the competence and integrity of many bodies, institutions, organizations, associations, foundations and companies. Not the individuals within them but the institutions themselves.

What we commonly believe about diet is not working. We have been conditioned to believe things about 'diet' that have nothing to do with health or well-being. Diet theories tend to be designed to promote certain products or 'food groups' and are based on 'science' that is frequently shallow or flawed. Many so-called 'experts' in diet cannot see the wood for the trees – others seek to mislead us deliberately for corporate interests.

There are good foods and there are bad 'foods'. Many things that we accept as 'food' are not food at all. When we know the difference it can change the way we think. When we change the way we think we change the way we behave. It is our behaviour that causes us to be fat, sick and tired.

The way we eat, think and move is largely responsible for how well we are. Many of the diseases that kill us are self-inflicted. Obesity, heart disease, diabetes, cancer, osteoporosis, depression, arthritis, allergies, and infertility might be termed 'diseases of choice' because they can be the natural consequence of poor decisions. The decisions are our responsibility, but we cannot be responsible if we are not properly informed. We are not well informed because there are groups of people who make it their business to ensure we continue to buy the products that make us sick, and then buy the products that ease our pain. Most of the sickness and pain can be avoided if we follow some simple guidelines, although they run much deeper than '5 portions of fruit and veg a day' or 'a healthy balanced diet'.

Livetetics raises some important issues for groups and for individuals. It is written with good intention. It is based on results. It works. I give it to you with the hope you will take from it what works for you. It has the potential to change lives, to extend lives and to improve lives. It is about life: your life; all our lives. That's why it is called 'LIVE'-tetics.

Livetetics is a summary of effective beliefs and experience. It is not 'right' or 'wrong'. Take it for what it is – a powerful observation of how things are and a proven way of transforming ourselves to the point of the perfection we deserve. At your fingertips is a pathway to energy, well-being, happiness and a fantastic-looking, healthy body. Look at the table below – it's a concise 'map' of the areas Livetetics will help you in the most.

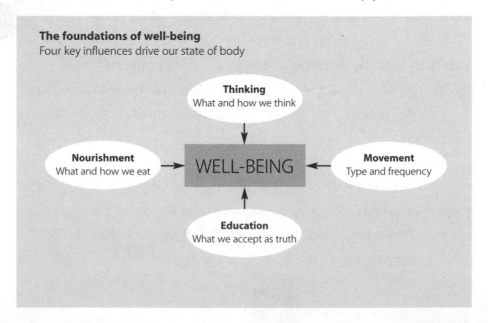

The foundations of well-being
Four key influences drive our state of body

Thinking
What and how we think

Nourishment
What and how we eat

WELL-BEING

Movement
Type and frequency

Education
What we accept as truth

Why do Livetetics?

Hello. I do not know you and you do not know me. However, we are intimately connected. We breathe the same air, we experience the same gravity, our sky shows the same moon, we experience the same sun. In fact, if you are more than 12 years old, no matter where on earth you live, it is almost certain that my body contains atoms that once were in your body and your body contains atoms that once were in mine.

Atoms are tiny, imperceptible bundles of energy. Everything is made of these little collections of matter. We take in billions of atoms every time we draw breath. We get rid of billions of different atoms every time we breathe out.

Your body is in a constant state of change and flux. As you breathe in, air is drawn into your lungs and some of it dissolves in your blood. This then goes on to feed and nourish cells in your body. The air literally becomes part of you. Every time you breathe out, atoms that were once part of your body are released from your blood into your lungs and you give them out, wherever you are.

The movement of this energy, these atoms, is totally impartial. A moment ago this energy was part of something else, now it is part of you. It stays part of you for a while, then it becomes part of something else. The atoms, this energy, care nothing for your politics, your size, your religion, your sex, your profession, your beliefs or your social standing. In every breath you share energy with people who are 'worse' than you and 'better' than you. You share it with animals, plants and insects.

While you have been reading so far you have probably inhaled atoms that were once part of Jesus, Mohammed, Mother Theresa, William Shakespeare, Henry VIII, Osama Bin Laden, Florence Nightingale, Jack the Ripper, Princess Diana and George Bush (in no particular order!).

Draw breath now. Notice it. Take a deep breath and stop for a moment to experience how it feels. Do it again. Breathe in billions of atoms. Breathe out billions of atoms. Every time you do this you make an exchange with your environment. You take some in and let some out. During the moments you have been reading you have shared atoms that were once part of the people around you right now (whether you like them or not!) and they have shared atoms with you. In this way you are in constant transition, always changing, sharing with the environment. You are part of me and I am part of you – we have no choice in the matter. Atoms that were once part of my skeleton, liver, skin, muscle may now be part of you and parts of you may now be part of me. So, like it not, we are connected. But I don't know you.

There are, however, some things I do know. I know for certain that you are a one-off. There are a billion aspects of your body, your experience, your life that make you unique. You have thoughts and aspirations that no-one else has. You know things that no-one else knows. You experience this world in a way that is totally individual to you and that no-one else will ever fully understand. There are things you don't understand and have given up trying to understand. There are things you do well, even brilliantly, yet there is still so much for you to learn about so many things.

Livetetics is about beliefs first. Our beliefs shape our decisions and our actions. You are already making decisions about this book, about me – these are based on your experiences so far in your life, on the way you look at things, on your interpretation of the way I use words and the beginnings of the presentation of my thoughts. I don't know how your beliefs are forming and how positive you feel about Livetetics right now. My hope, of course, is that you have some emerging interest and curiosity to find out what Livetetics is all about.

Beliefs are very important – you are about to find out how important they are and why so many people are after you for your beliefs. I urge you to approach Livetetics with an open mind. For some, this is a very difficult thing to do. Some people believe they are right and will do anything to discount or ignore evidence that upsets that view.

It is fine for you not to believe me. You do not have to accept that Livetetics is true or that its strategies work brilliantly. The only way for you to assess the effectiveness of Livetetics is to live the Livetetic way for 90 days and let the results help you decide.

I run a well-being consulting network, from which Livetetics was born. One of the services offered by that network is an online health and well-being profile that gives people tailored advice about how to lose weight. People complete a detailed questionnaire about their symptoms, lifestyle and what they eat and, based on their profile, we then offer simple recommendations for the most important changes they need to make.

As part of the ongoing process we regularly review feedback from clients to see what does and doesn't work for people. We strive to find out how we can make things even better. We send out questionnaires, interview clients and make sure we review and record all letters of comment, thanks and complaint.

Something struck us one day when reviewing unsolicited letters of congratulations and complaint we received from people who had purchased an online profile. Bear in mind that the online service delivers a recommended diet and supplement programme to be followed for 90 days (three months) before reassessment.

It was the timing of the letters that was so striking. All the complaints came within 24 hours of the profile being generated. They said things like:

'This advice is too obvious. I could read this in any women's magazine.'

'You recommended that I should take food supplements and I don't agree with supplementation.'

'The advice that I should eat much less wheat and dairy is too impractical and, anyway, dairy foods are an important food group.'

The congratulations and thanks however would come much later; three, six or nine months after purchasing the profile. Quotes from these people included:

'Thank you. After 15 years of trying every diet I have finally lost weight for good.'

'It is amazing. Not only have I lost weight but my energy has gone through the roof and my joint pain has disappeared.'

'For the first time in 10 years I can walk and sit without pain in my hips.'

'Thank you so much. I did what you said and I feel so much better. All my friends have noticed the change and ask what I've been doing.'

So what is the difference between the complainers and the successes?

The fact is that the complainers never even tried it. They read the report and did nothing – except complain – usually because they had received something they didn't expect and didn't believe would work. These are the type of people who complain about their pain, their bodies, their cellulite, their headaches, their bad relationships – but never do anything different to make things better, even when they can, so easily.

On the other hand, the successes did try. They simply did. And they succeeded. By making the required changes they found a new path, got rewarded along the way and kept going.

Think for a moment about the person who inspires you most.

We have all experienced someone in our lives who inspired us to do something that made us feel much better. Think of that person now. What was it that they did that encouraged you to make the change: to make that positive move; to do that crazy thing; to wear that outrageous outfit; to visit that amazing place; to make that call? How good did it feel?

I know who that person was. I know who it was that encouraged you to do the greatest thing you've ever done. I also know who is stopping you from doing the things you know you could do right now to make it much, much better. You know who this person is. But how well do you know them?

Welcome to yourself

Only you can inspire yourself. Things people say, things you read, experiences you have – all play a part in shaping your decisions but it is only you that makes the decisions and takes the action.

How easy could it be for you to take the actions you need to look and feel your best? Just how quickly could you be inspired to raise your head above the misinformation in our society, to breathe clean fresh air and see how amazing life can be? When you do you'll smell the sweet, pure scent of reality over fiction. When you lift your head and look through the fog, as your vision clears you will notice things you hadn't noticed before.

We often look but don't see. We often listen but don't hear. We often know what to **do but don't** do what we know.

There is **only one** way for you to know how effective Livetetics is. And that is to live it. **Why do it?** To regain total well-being.

I wish you well. You are about to embark on a journey to a new place. It is a place you always dreamed of. You know the place. It lives in your imagination. A place where you are everything you ever wanted to be, where you feel strong inside, totally comfortable and ready for anything, a place where you can be yourself and nothing else matters. People look at you in a new way, a way that makes you feel good inside, a good feeling that grows and allows you to take on new ideas and do things you never thought you would do. A place where you are in control, you call the shots and nothing can stop you being the person you deserve to be. Perfect in every way. Relax and feel comfortable and strong in the knowledge that you are in control and are ready to do what works for you and only what works for you.

Do it for 90 days – and then judge Livetetics.

The battle for our beliefs

BELIEFS – WHY WE THINK THE WAY WE DO

The world is full of uncertainty. Is the earth round or flat? You should believe it to be round. We've all heard about the astronomer called Galileo who first claimed it to be so, and who spent his life being ridiculed by the establishment as a result. Galileo's peers thought he was mad, a heretic, a lunatic. The 'experts' of the day believed the earth was flat and that dreadful things would happen to you if you fell off the edge. The notion that the earth was round was incredible, ridiculous, beggared belief and was just plain nonsense. In the end the round-earthers won their argument and we now, generally, believe that the earth is round. But how do you know the earth is round? Have you, personally, left the earth in a spaceship and looked back and seen it?

So, how can you be sure the earth is round? You can't see it's round from where you're standing. You can't tell it's round from a plane as you fly to the other side of it. Your parents told you it's round when you were a tiny tot. You were taught at school that it's round. You've seen pictures that other people have told you were taken from space. The whole establishment tells you now that the earth is round. But what if it were all a con? What if it were all a fabrication to prevent you from finding out what happened at the edge?

Imagine for a moment that your school teachers were just teaching you what they had been taught to teach you – they had no reason to know they were teaching you a pack of lies but they believed the writers of the text books. What if the astronomers, geographers and physicists had made a dreadful, incredible mistake and it turned out that they were wrong. Imagine if the space pictures weren't real at all but were just computer-generated mock ups created to give the impression that a space ship had left the earth and taken photographs of a spherical planet.

Would it be possible for the world's population to be conned into such an idea?

How might you react to such a proposition? The notion that this spherical earth confidence trick could be occurring defies the imagination; it is just plain nonsense. These were exactly the reactions of Galileo's peers when he dared to rock the status quo.

Now I am not postulating that the earth is round or that it is flat. I am only confirming that I cannot know that either of these is true without taking a lot of my references on trust. I am sure that if I spent some time with astronomers and used a telescope I would gain more references for my beliefs one way or the other. But I could never really be certain until I actually experienced it. And so it is with a great many beliefs.

By their early teens most people have a lot of belief baggage that holds them back. We have a tendency to trust and respect authority figures – our parents, our teachers, doctors, the media, independent 'experts', spokespeople. Over time we create belief systems that help us live in our environment. There are things we believe to be 'true', things we believe are 'facts' and things that we believe are 'real'.

Your views might be different to mine. So which of us is correct? You or I? Should you listen to me or should I listen to you?

The answer is, of course, that only by listening fully to one another do we stand any chance of knowing more. What Livetetics is all about is offering you the opportunity to free yourself of the baggage of your beliefs. It is, after all, your beliefs that drive your actions and that is why they are so valuable. Your beliefs are probably your most prized

Any 'fact' that you have not discovered for yourself is something you take on trust. Be careful – even people you trust can have very poor beliefs. Be especially careful of 'experts'; they are often the most dangerous of all

possessions and that is why so many people are after you for them.

Try answering the questions below. Write a list – two columns – positives on the left and negatives on the right. Consider for a moment why you make these decisions for and about yourself.

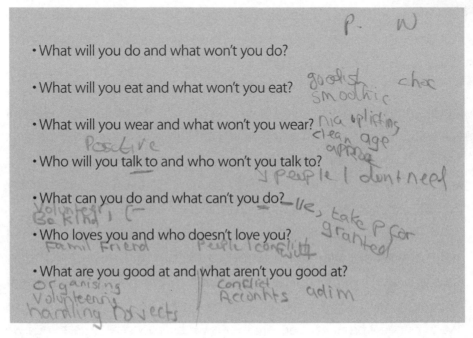

• What will you do and what won't you do?

• What will you eat and what won't you eat?

• What will you wear and what won't you wear?

• Who will you talk to and who won't you talk to?

• What can you do and what can't you do?

• Who loves you and who doesn't love you?

• What are you good at and what aren't you good at?

You might like to try another important exercise. Some people hate exercises in books so feel free to leave this out but, just in case you are minded to learn something, fill in the following grids. It is a good limbering-up exercise to start flexing your belief-system muscles. Beliefs need to be exercised, stretched, renewed, challenged and sometimes discarded when necessary. Most of us just leave a lot of beliefs intact for no good reason. Others are worth hanging on to and these should be kept in pride of place and well polished.

List opposite five things that you know absolutely to be true. Next to each one write down the evidence you have that proves it is true. We're after five rock-solid beliefs.

Absolute Truth	How I know this to be true
1. my Boy love me	I Just know, N1 & alway we say it - Both ways touch feudd le very NB
2. Very good things come t a rind	Er perir of holidays sheual find mov on Relations end - death A lovely mead
3. Ailing Business Can only go on for so long	→ I am it
4. I am a very busy persn and know it t need it "	It get commend on " " praise on certain people need to be . It does t hav to PA10 to busy
5. I have realised L dont have a real relationship with my famil.	→ lifetime of Experur = Different level of contked - difficult hame Parent -- sliting oo very deep

This exercise is one of the most important aspects of living Livetetics. Testing out your beliefs is a great way of discarding limiting and unwanted constraints. The column on the right – how you know each thing to be true – is crucial. These are the references you use to support your beliefs. If we think of our beliefs as table tops then the references are the legs that hold a belief up for us.

So a belief like:

Absolute Truth	How I know this to be true
I have ten fingers	I can see them, I can count them, I use them every day, I am looking at them now.

... is a pretty strong belief. It's based on very solid references.

Look at the belief below:

Absolute Truth	How I know this to be true
I am a failure	I haven't achieved what I wanted in life. Other people have more than me. I'm fat and don't feel good. I can never stick to a diet. Compared with the people I read about I haven't achieved nearly enough.

This is no less solid for many people than 'I have ten fingers'. But the references are much more shaky. They are subjective references and subject to interpretation and comparison with things that may or may not be real.

The 'I am a failure' belief is almost universally held (believe it or not). When I work with clients, most of them believe they are failures. A famous rock musician believes he is a failure in love and relationships and would trade all his money and fame for them. A career woman who has made an enormous success of her businesses feels a failure as a wife and mother because she is not home as much as she feels she ought to be. A fantastic mother in a happy relationship feels unfulfilled and a failure for not having a career. A superb schoolteacher, who loves his work, feels a failure because he hasn't found a way to apply his passion and talent in a way that will buy him a decent house or car.

Notice that the 'I am a failure' belief has a lot of references that are based not on actual fact but on a perception of how things 'ought' to be, could be, might be – 'If only I were truly successful'. There are beliefs that are based on reality and beliefs that are based on perceptions of reality: unfortunately we all tend to be rather hard on ourselves.

Go back to your five beliefs on page 25 and look critically at your references. Underline the references that you absolutely, personally KNOW to be true because you have experienced them, seen them yourself or can test them for yourself. You will find that many of your beliefs are based on very shallow references – the opinion of your parents, what you were taught at school, what some group of 'experts' believes or what some journalist or TV producer puts out.

Try the exercise again, this time with some attributes about yourself.

Trust me, this is important. This book isn't called 'Read and Grow Thin' – a better title would be 'Change and Look Better', 'Do and Feel Better', 'Adjust and Get More Comfortable'. It is only by doing some different things that you will get a different result. Livetetics is about permanent shifts in thinking and behaviour. And Livetetics is about results. If you do it you succeed. If you don't, you won't.

So, start with five positive attributes about yourself, things that you know absolutely to be true. Choose anything: I am alive. I can think. I can breathe. I can read. I can change. I am beautiful. I am sexy. I am intelligent. I am wise. I am a great lover. I am a great father/mother. I am a wonderful friend. I am in complete control. I am… whatever you love most about yourself and your life. Think of some and write them down over the page.

> *It is only by doing different things that you can get different results*

Absolute Truth	How I know this to be true
1.	
2.	
3.	
4.	
5.	

Play with this exercise a little. When you think you've taken it as far as you think you can, try it again, only this time with things you think about yourself that are not positive. Again, my experience with clients is that people find it much easier to make a list of negative attributes than positive ones. BUT – the references for the positive tend to be much stronger than the negative.

So people might say things like: I am a failure, I am fat, I can never stick to anything, I am lazy, I am shy, I am a loser, I am scared, I am depressed, I am stupid, I am bad, I am mean, I am poor, I am weak, I am a bad speaker. Most negative self-beliefs come from interpretations of past experiences, things people said or didn't say or self-imposed perceptions of how things ought to be.

One of my clients told me this story. Jane was five. She was a little unsure about school and one day her teacher asked everyone in the class to stand up and say something about their weekend. Jane really didn't want to do this. She spent the next half hour absolutely dreading the calling of her name. She felt sick. When her name was called she almost froze but was eventually persuaded to stand up. Everything was a blur. Her teacher cajoled and questioned and teased some words out of her. Some of the class laughed and sniggered. Jane was mortified, shocked, humiliated. This experience left the child with some limiting beliefs about her 'shyness', 'poor speaking ability' and 'lack of presence' or 'confidence'.

In fact the only belief Jane needed was that she had an incompetent teacher who should have found a better way to help her feel confident and comfortable enough to speak freely to her class. The teacher should have known better. This is a very common issue. Fear of public speaking is one of the most common problems or worries I come across and almost invariably it comes down to a couple of bad classroom experiences induced by well-meaning yet incompetent teachers. Most people never learn to sing for exactly the same reason. The good news is that this and other limiting beliefs can be changed in a heartbeat: if you know how.

It's the diet, not you

Some people believe they can never stick to a diet, that they have a lack of willpower and that this makes them fat. The references they provide include listing endless forays into calorie-controlled diets, faddy diets and attendance at weigh-in sessions where they are encouraged week by week to count food in points or calories and then feel guilty or a failure when it is unsustainable and they don't succeed. While we do have a responsibility to ourselves in making the best of any decisions we make, this 'failure' actually says nothing about the person: it is simply evidence of the inadequacy of the regime they were trying. So here's a suggestion; why not blame the diet?

It's difficult to blame the diet; after all there is so much 'evidence' that people do succeed on the regime. The papers talk about celebrities that succeed. The weight-loss club magazine tells monthly stories about women who lose so much weight by following their rules. Every week someone is congratulated for losing the most weight that week. It MUST be possible!

It is interesting to note that most diet clubs rely significantly on repeat business. That is, they rely on people that come back year after year to try and lose weight. If the diets worked – surely they would be lean by now? It's weird really – most businesses rely on selling a quality product to gain loyalty from their customers. The diet industry on the other hand sells a product that doesn't work and people end up going back and back and back for more.

Things are, very often, not what they seem.

Testing your references

Listed opposite and below are a few common beliefs. Go quickly through each one and decide whether the statement is true or false. Tick the box and move on. Ignore the references for now.

Then add up all your True and False answers.

Belief	True	False	References
There is no such thing as an unhealthy food, only an unhealthy diet		✓	
Pharmaceutical medicines (drugs) are the main factors in improving human health and lifespan		✓	
A little alcohol (especially red wine) is beneficial to your health	✓		
Legal food additives have been proven safe	✓		
Small quantities of pesticides in your food will do you no harm		✓	
The government food guidelines are based on independent science and full understanding of food and health		✓	
Refined sugar is a food and a source of healthy energy		✓	
The government cares about your health and actively seeks prevention of unnecessary diseases		✓	
There is a difference between 'artificial' and 'natural' flavourings	✓		
Crisps are safe for children to eat	✓		
Sugar is not an addictive drug		✓	

Belief	True	False	References
Taking licensed medications is always safe			
Nuts and seeds are fattening			
Food law will protect you from corrupt manufacturers			
Advertising to children doesn't influence them			
You need to eat meat to be healthy			
Vegetarian diets are always healthier than meat eating diets			
You can get all the nutrients you need from a 'healthy balanced diet'			
Fruit sold as fresh is fresh			
Organic foods are healthy			
Food supplements are unnecessary if you eat well			
Any food proven to make people ill would be taken off the market			
Foods known to cause obesity and disease would have to carry health warnings			

Belief	True	False	References
The government RDAs (Recommended Daily Allowance) for vitamins and minerals are based on what you need to be optimally healthy	✓		
We already have the knowledge and resources to virtually eradicate cancer		✓	
You can catch a cold		✓	
Chemical medicines (drugs) can cure diseases	✓		
Official and statutory bodies of diet and nutrition are independent		✓	
Heart disease is inevitable for some people	✓		
The government guideline for salt intake is safe		✓	
Taking more than the RDA of vitamins and minerals is worthless	✓		
Pharmaceutical companies care primarily about your health		✓	
Disease in old age is inevitable	✓		

Belief	True	False	References
The increase in degenerative diseases (heart disease, cancer, diabetes) is mainly because we are getting older as a population		✓	
Schools are obliged to feed children food that is healthy and safe		✓	
If foods were identified as potential killers they would be removed from the market		✓	
Your genes play a large part in whether you are fat or not	✓		
Your genes dictate your health		✓	
You can trust your doctor to take the best care of your health		✓	
National Health Services need more money		✓	
Your doctor is obliged to warn you about side effects of medicines		✓	
Government funded health services look for and use the most effective treatments		✓	
If there were natural cures for killer diseases we would know about them		✓	

Belief	True	False	References
Milk is good for you and dairy products are an essential part of a healthy diet – especially for children	✓		
If the government knew of common nutrient deficiencies in our children they would help to solve the problem	✓		
If confectionery/sweets were proved dangerous they would no longer be sold to children	✓		
The people who make the laws about food fully understand nutrition and health	✓		
The people who make the laws about medicines act in the interest of the public	✓		
Independent health charities have been set up to improve research into diseases and look for cures	✓		
Lack of exercise is the major reason our children are getting increasingly obese and unhealthy	✓		
Heat treated, packaged fruit juices have the same nutritional benefits as fresh, raw juices		✓	

Belief	True	False	References
A tin of skimmed milk containing 8 spoons of sugar and 1/3 the RDA of vitamins and minerals is a healthy meal replacement		✓	
A carton of sugar water containing 10 spoons of sugar, 5 per cent 'real juice' and is 'rich in Vitamin C' is a healthy drink for a child		✓	
'Perfectly Balanced' when written on a food label in a major supermarket means the food is healthy and will contribute to your well-being		✓	
All calories are equal. There is no difference in the calories from a chocolate biscuit or a piece of fresh apple		✓	
A bottle of sugar water containing as much as 15 teaspoons of sugar, orange colouring and a tiny amount of vitamins is an effective source of energy		✓	
Going on a diet is the only effective way to lose weight		✓	
Arthritis is best treated with anti-inflammatory drugs		✓	
Depression is best treated with anti-depressant drugs		✓	

Belief	True	False	References
ADHD children have a disease that needs drug treatment		✓	
Genetically Modified food can be proven safe to grow and eat		✓	

	True	False
Total		

If you scored more than 45 as true then you will benefit enormously from a change in your belief systems. If you scored more than 45 as false then you have already been limbering up your belief systems and you are well on your way to freedom from fat, physical degeneration and disease.

According to Livetetics experience and principles, all of these statements are, for the most part, false. More will be explained later. If you find the statements here true then you are falling victim to a set of beliefs that are not optimizing your health and well-being. Go back and take a look at your answers and consider the references you have for each belief. If you don't have a strong set of self-references for the statement – that is, you have personally seen or experienced evidence that it is true – then deem it false for now and make a note not to take this statement for granted in future. Most of these questions are a latent 'True' for most people. They aren't particularly questions you might ask yourself directly but they are very, very important.

It is a sad truth that the environment of beliefs about food is so riddled with misunderstanding, confusion and industry propaganda that we are literally digging our graves with our teeth.

Knowledge is, indeed, power

The fantastic news is that once you start to acknowledge this you will find changes much easier to make. Once you understand the root cause of what is compromising the way you look and feel, it then becomes so much easier to make better decisions.

We live in an environment where our beliefs are very important – particularly so to other people and organizations who seek to benefit from our decisions and actions. Our beliefs are important to the government because they want us to live in an orderly way and pay our taxes. They are important to big companies and industries because they want us to keep buying their products and not question how those products are produced, or to what cost. They are important for parents because they want the best for us and they want us to be all they wanted to be. They are important for children because they just want to be loved.

Our beliefs are shaped by people and things around us: our parents, teachers, doctors, newspapers, television, radio, magazines, books, friends, enemies, ministers. It is time to stop relying on the outside world for your belief system. Your beliefs are precious. We owe it to ourselves to base our beliefs only on what we know to be true despite this truth being sometimes strange and hard to find.

Livetetics does not presume to be a philosophy. It is simply a collection of empowering beliefs that have been created and, based on experience rather than manipulated science, shown to work. They are not beliefs created by the suppression of evidence that creates confusion and conflict; they are not based on any self-serving outcome and they are not based on frequent advertising or public relations activity.

Livetetics is based on results. Livetetics gets results. Livetetics is a results-oriented way of living. Do NOT take my word for it. Just do it – then decide for yourself.

WHY WE CARE – WHY NOT STAY JUST AS WE ARE?

S it up straight. Take a deep breath (count slowly to five as you do). Hold it for a few seconds (count slowly to five). And exhale slowly (count to ten as you do).

Do this 5–10 times, each time a little deeper. Absolutely fill your lungs and then completely empty them.

Fantastic. Pay attention to your fingers and how they feel. Take one more really deep breath and see how long it takes to notice the effect it has in your fingers. You might notice feelings elsewhere as well. Become conscious of your breathing and the energy it brings you. As the atoms in each breath race to the furthest reaches of your body they bring refreshment, energy and change.

Since you started reading this chapter, cells in your body have died and grown. Atoms in every corner of your body have come and gone. Your entire body is in a constant state of change and flux. Notice it. You can feel it if you pay attention. Your skin is regenerating all the time. Your skeleton is constantly rebuilding; your kidneys are breaking down and reforming as are all your organs – your liver, your heart, your intestines. All of these things are changing, constantly regenerating. And we must help our bodies as much as we can to carry out this process cleanly, economically and healthily.

Breathing air in a tube train is different to breathing air in an open field. Breathing air in the office is different to breathing it outside. Breathing just after you have sprayed your underarm with deodorant has a different effect than breathing at an open window.

> *The body you have now is different from the body you had when you started reading this chapter*

> *Your life.*
> *Your choice.*
> *Your decision.*

Deciding how deeply to breathe, and at what pace, and finding places where it feels good to breathe all make a difference to the way you feel, how energized you are, how efficiently your bodily processes work, how you look and how well you are.

If you want oxygen in your skin, breathing is the best way to get it there. Some people have created a belief that they can get it there by applying patented skin creams containing oxygen. I recommend you stick with breathing, save your money and enjoy healthier skin.

Your beliefs drive your decisions. Your decisions drive your actions. Your actions drive your destiny.

You are constantly making decisions. To do the exercises in this book or not to do the exercises in this book. To take a deep breath or not to take a deep breath. To now sit upright, relax your shoulders, hold the book up and gently stretch your head upwards away from your hips so you feel a nice long stretch in your spine. Or not to bother.

How to sit, how to stand, where to go, who to talk to, what to eat, what to drink, how to breathe. All your decisions affect how you are. Livetetics is very simple really. It's about making better decisions.

I'm afraid that staying just as you are isn't an option. You are changing. Like it or not you are changing, every moment, with every heartbeat, with every breath. You are changing, regenerating. And the nature of these changes and this regeneration is largely up to you. You have the potential to be in control of both your mental and physical well-being.

This is very good news. It places you in total control of yourself and your life, and gives you freedom to change pretty much whatever you want very quickly. It brings responsibility as well. Responsibility for your health, well-being and how you look and feel. We are all, for the most part, individually responsible for how well and vital we are. Vitality, well-being and a perfect body do not come from pills or creams, doctors or gurus.

Perfect health and a great body come from the little actions we take moment to moment – it starts with your next breath.

So whether or not you do a single thing that is recommended in Livetetics, you are making decisions that will affect your outcome. What will your body be like in a year, or ten years from now? How will you feel?

It is worth thinking about. Most of the people that walk through my door wanting to look and feel better tend to tell me about all the things they don't want. But you have to set a goal if you are to achieve change.

'I want to get rid of this fat'

'I don't want this cellulite'

'I don't want to be depressed all the time'

'I want to get rid of my headaches and mood swings'

'I want to stop feeling bad'

'I want to stop feeling a failure'

'I need to eat less chocolate and junk'

It is much more powerful – and you are more likely to achieve success – to decide how you want things to be rather than how you don't want them to be. Rather than the negative statements above, a more positive way of setting your targets or goals would be:

'I want my tummy to be flat and my arms and legs to be lean

and shapely'

'I would like my skin to be smooth and supple and have great colour'

'I want to feel happy and upbeat all the time'

'I want to feel clear headed, comfortable and friendly all day'

'I want to feel wonderful about everything'

'I want to feel that I am successful'

'I would like to eat more positive foods'

When my clients start to set clear and specific targets for what they actually want to achieve, they start to achieve them much more quickly and easily.

Just for a moment consider what it is you want to achieve. When you picked up Livetetics, what was it you wanted to get from it? What did you hope to achieve?

Opposite is a table for you to fill in. I make no apologies for making you work! It is too easy to read books or articles and, no matter how much of a chord they strike, to then go away and make no changes to your life. With these tables I aim to get you thinking, really thinking, perhaps for the first time in your life.

> *You cannot hit a target you cannot see. You cannot reach a goal you do not have.*

Think now, and write down how your life will be when it is the way you want it to be. In your head, start each sentence with:

'When I am the way I want to be and everything is perfect…'

How will I feel when I wake in the morning?	
How much energy will I have?	
What will my body reflect when I see it in the mirror?	
What will I say to myself about my body?	
How will I feel when I sit down for a quiet moment?	
What clothes will I wear?	
What things will I do for pleasure?	
What great relationships will I have?	
What will I say to myself about what I have achieved?	

Well done. This is a great start. This is something we all need to keep doing every few months or so, to assess and reassess how we are doing. Our priorities and ideas about what we want change all the time. But to have a constant picture, a clear description and a positive feeling about exactly where we are going and what we are doing is perhaps the most important thing we can do. Go into as much detail as you can.

What will my body reflect when I see it in the mirror?	There will be a smiling face that is lit up and my eyes will sparkle. My hair will be in great condition. My shoulders will be relaxed and look strong with my arms lean. My tummy will be as firm as it can be and my legs will be lean and strong. My skin will glow with healthy colour and it will be strong and supple. My body will look younger than it does now and some of my youthful looks will have returned. Overall I will look fabulous and I will feel fabulous about it.

Above is a real goal from a real person who came to me with the original objective of getting rid of cellulite on her thighs. She was considering liposuction. She was depressed, had been on endless diets and just felt bad about her life and her looks. She had considerable difficulty even thinking about her body in a positive way.

It is important, as you gradually improve and hone your aims, to think about yourself as you set goals. Don't aspire to be somebody else. Be free to feel good about yourself, just as you are, and then imagine feeling even better about yourself just as you are. What are held up as today's icons of beauty, well-being, cool or good looks, are simply products of fashion. Fashion changes – be yourself.

Focus first on feelings

When we embark on a process of change to improve how we look the temptation is to become unduly concerned about the physical manifestation of the change rather than how we want to feel. It is a clear Livetetic belief that it is by first changing how we feel that we will be able to change how we behave.

It is a common mistake to think that when something happens then, and only then, will we feel better.

For example:

> 'When I have lost a stone then I will feel better'
>
> 'When I can get into my jeans then I'll feel good'
>
> 'When my belly doesn't hang over my belt – then I'll feel better'

We will learn that this is the wrong way around. It is by feeling better first that the changes come more easily. A lot of our negative behaviour comes from unhelpful beliefs, but it also comes from not feeling as good as we'd like to. Eating certain foods can change the way we feel. They change the chemistry in our bodies and can give the illusion of making us feel better for a period of time. They create biochemical and physiological changes that trick us into believing they make us feel good. For the most part these 'foods' are 'mentally' addictive and, physically, are actually having the opposite effect to the one we are 'feeling'.

If you experience cravings for certain foods the craving is usually for returning your body to the way it was before you started eating the food in the first place. The craving can be seen as a chemical illusion.

Cravings for foods are often just signals that your body wants to return to feeling the way it did before you ate that food. This can be the root of addiction to unhelpful 'foods'

Smoking

It is the same as smoking. The smoker smokes to feel better. But that good feeling is really an illusion. Smokers crave cigarettes so that they can feel the way they would feel if they were non-smokers. Smoking messes up the body's chemistry so that smokers only feel 'normal' if they are smoking. The craving for the cigarette is the body trying to feel the way it used to feel before the smoking habit started. Smokers actually spend their money and lives trying to feel the way they would if they weren't smoking at all. Yet they continue to believe, congruently, that smoking makes them feel good, and in spite of the certain knowledge that they are killing themselves they continue the habit.

This is the sad reality going on around us. Statistically, three quarters of us will die of a degenerative disease. Degenerative diseases include things like cancer, heart disease and diabetes. These are diseases that are created by the breakdown of parts of our body or of normal body processes, and an inability by the body to regenerate itself perfectly or efficiently, which is often due to the way we live and the choices we make.

It is now undisputed that smoking kills people, thanks to this degenerative/regenerative issue. But in spite of warnings, in stark letters on cigarette packets, people continue to do it. Why?

Smokers have been conned. They have been conned initially into thinking smoking delivers something to them that justifies the expense of doing it. For many it begins with a need to show bravado, to look cool or to demonstrate emergence from childhood into adulthood. It starts, for most, as a social statement. It is normally quite unpleasant to begin with but, with perseverance, people learn to suck the smoke from the burning leaves into their lungs and ignore the burning, rasping, cutting pain it creates in their throat and the sick nauseous feeling it induces.

The ace up the cigarette's sleeve, of course, is that it contains an addictive drug. A drug that alters the way the smoker feels. Smoking, overall, actually makes people feel terrible. It has the effect of making them stressed, irritable and nervous. The act of smoking, though, delivers an addictive drug that temporarily suppresses the bad feelings that smoking creates. It's a vicious cycle. So the smoker is on a continual quest to feel like a non-smoker – the way they did before they started smoking. Smokers believe that the relief of smoking is worth the price – not just the cost of the cigarettes but the dramatically increased probability of ghastly painful death from an unnecessary disease that will destroy them and their loved ones. The reality is they pay a fortune and give their lives just to feel the way they would if they hadn't started smoking in the first place.

It is extraordinary, isn't it?

Increases in childhood disease

I spoke a few years ago with a respected doctor in The Hague in Holland. He had practised medicine during the 1960s and 70s. His son was now a doctor too and was practising in a children's ward where he, the father, had worked many years before. The older man recounted a series of visits to his son in the hospital where there were children with leukaemia, heart problems and other degenerative disorders. He recalled his own time at the hospital and how these sorts of problems were so rare when he was a younger man. He told me how sad he was that in the last 40 years we had managed to create a society where our children were sicker now than they have ever been.

His concerns are playing out everywhere. We have skyrocketing rates of childhood obesity. Late-onset diabetes, usually typical of adults, is now becoming apparent in children. Childhood heart conditions are on the rise, as are cancers and immune deficiency diseases. The autistic spectrum disorders from ADHD and autism through to more chronic mental disorders are also increasing.

What's going on?

Our modern medical system is akin to a brave walker who hears a cry for help from a person in a river. The walker rushes to the riverbank to see someone struggling for breath in the water. He dives in without regard for his own safety and swims over to rescue the drowning individual. He swims back to the bank, drags the unfortunate person out of the water and begins to resuscitate them. No sooner does the poor, wet person start to cough back into consciousness than our intrepid rescuer hears another person's cry from the river. So he dives in again and performs yet another heroic rescue.

After getting the second person into recovery he hears, this time, two cries. There are two more victims in the river – he screams for help and calls for support. As he carries the two back to shore he is joined by another walker who happens to be passing. Together they resuscitate the individuals and try to keep the others warm – but no sooner are they through than there are more cries from the direction of the river.

Exhausted, they continue rescuing, always having to dive in and help again before they are even able to catch their breath.

If only they could find time to run upriver and find out what is causing the people to fall in.

And so it is with our health services. They are set up to rescue us and they do a marvellous job. But when it comes to the degenerative diseases, they just haven't got round to stopping us from falling in the river. Self-inflicted diseases: like smokers, most of us are addicted to lifestyles and diets that are killing us. It is really showing in our children.

We, largely, are personally responsible for:

being fat,

being tired,

being depressed,

being impotent,

having bad skin,

looking baggy and droopy

and developing heart disease,

arthritis,

osteoporosis,

cancer and

diabetes

I know that avoiding these diseases isn't a very compelling reason for making changes – any danger of them is always in the future, or going to happen to someone else. They are something we don't want, but don't really do much to actively avoid.

Over the years, I have learned that people largely get what they focus on. So in Livetetics we focus on what we do want. Let's remind ourselves of the thing that Livetetics can deliver:

a lean, beautiful body,

being full of energy,

feeling great,

youthful skin,

looking fabulous in your pants,

a strong healthy heart,

flexible, comfortable joints,

strong muscles and bones,

freedom from disease and

an excellent sex life

WHOM SHOULD WE LISTEN TO?

It is so important to be careful about whom and what we believe. It is essential that we make sure our references are solid.

Parents are not necessarily right just because they are parents. Teachers are not necessarily right just because they are teachers. Dieticians are not necessarily right just because they are dieticians. The chief medical officer is not necessarily right just because he is the chief medical officer. The weight-loss club is not necessarily right just because it has been in business for decades and has a lot of members. Livetetics is not necessarily right just because I say it works.

The parent who gives a child a sweet, sugared drink thinking it gives him or her energy does so not out of ignorance, but with a belief that the drink will give energy.

The teacher who encourages a child to eat up everything on their plate does so, not out of ignorance, but because of a belief that it will be helpful for the child.

The doctors who prescribe a drug for a nutrition-related condition do so because they believe it is the right thing to do.

The dieticians who encourage all mothers to include milk and dairy products in their children's diets do so because their education delivers a belief that this is the best thing to do.

And the chief medical officer who presides over a health system that predominantly acts as a distribution channel for drugs and medical equipment rather than acting to prevent unnecessary diseases does so, not because of back-handers from manufacturers, but because of a belief that it is in the public interest.

A great many well-intentioned people have beliefs that are not helpful. The road to hell, as they say, is paved with good intentions.

Open your mind

Livetetics is not about being cynical and angry and not trusting anyone. It is purely about having an open mind, being receptive to better ideas and being much more self-reliant when making decisions. It is about using internal references (our own – how we actually look and feel) rather than external references (those that others suggest we should accept).

Next time you are sitting in a grassy place on a sunny day and you see a line of ants busying from one place to another, watch them for a while. Notice how they move rapidly yet precisely. Wonder at how they manage to lift objects sometimes two or three times their size over what, to them, are huge obstacles – blades of grass, twigs and the like. After you have been surprised at how they know where they are going, have marvelled at the way they are coordinated and help one another, and have wondered at how their community must be organized, then try this simple yet interesting experiment.

On one side of the line of ants sprinkle the crumbs from a crushed-up chocolate biscuit. On the other side of the line of ants sprinkle some broken fresh raw nuts and sunflower seeds.

Then sit and wait. Watch the ants and see what happens...

They will detour to the nuts and seeds and do anything they can to carry them back home. The crumbs from the biscuit will be left and won't be touched until all of the nuts and seeds have been recovered. I have never seen the ants take the biscuit rather than the nuts and seeds.

Try it again. This time use a fresh strawberry that you have pinched between your fingers; place this on one side and a teaspoon of strawberry jam on the other. You guessed it, the ants go for the fresh strawberry. They pile on it in a huge bunch. They queue up to get to it. The jam will be left.

Ants are pretty smart. They will take whole grains of rice and they will pick up wholegrain flour but leave refined grains (white flour) and sugar.

I think that most of us would generally accept that raw nuts and fresh fruit are a better choice than a chocolate biscuit, a blob of jam or a spoonful of sugar. Yet people, when given the choice, will more often than not go for the wrong items.

There are no fat ants!

The ants are making a natural choice between 'live' foods and 'dead' foods. They can tell what is food – food that will provide good, healthy energy (see page 132 for what I mean by 'good' energy) and what is junk. How is it that an ant can make a better decision than a person?

The ants are unencumbered and live by their instinct. We, on the other hand, are largely divorced from our natural senses. We have become detached from the day-to-day choices we would have to make to survive in the wild and have become

Junk is valueless, negative material

dependent on institutions and organizations for our survival. We are mostly taught what to think rather than learning from self-experience: 'the earth is round, it is not flat'.

This ability, to learn from others, to amass history and experience, has been significantly responsible for the 'progress' of people in the way we build, create and organize. If we were able to ensure that the passage of knowledge from one generation to the next was entirely constructive then, I believe, we would solve virtually every issue of conflict and disease in the world. This would be the Livetetic way.

But we have made it much more complex than that. The way our society is structured means that we are largely dependent on external cues to determine how we feel. We have aspirations, but we want things we don't need, we eat things we don't need to eat, we compare ourselves with others and we listen, too much, to the advice of others.

I know of people who, for years, have been taking advice about health (and about their weight) from fat advisers – partners, doctors or friends. Why would any sane person do that? If you are fat and want to lose weight then why would you take advice from someone who clearly doesn't know how to do it?

This is a primary issue. Do not take advice from people who cannot demonstrate success. If you are going to take health advice you must take it from someone with a lean body, sparkling eyes, great skin and a cheery, friendly disposition. The sort of person that makes you feel better before you have even said 'hello'. But we don't do this. We are more impressed by the certificate on the wall, the white coat, the technology. These are the references and evidence we use to determine that the individual is able to give us useful advice.

And so it goes on. When a respected, well-spoken professor in a senior government post is interviewed on the television, people will accept what he says as true, for the most part. We have been sledge-hammered into respecting people all our lives: parents, teachers, doctors, ministers…

The media largely sets the national agenda. Have you ever wondered why, with all the newspapers, radio stations and television channels, the same big news item appears everywhere on the same day? We live in a world with a couple of hundred countries and six billion people but the main international news item will be the same on virtually every news broadcast. You find it all the time.

The reality is that the majority of what we hear, read and see on our radios, in our newspapers and on our televisions is often carefully orchestrated. It is telling us what is news and then what to think about it. The church was once used for this kind of mass communication. To encourage people that the poor would be rich in the after-life and to be happy with their lot. To be good, law-abiding citizens and to help one another. A useful message if you were a king who wished to keep the peasantry in its place and stop them wanting too much. Not to say, of course, that being a law abiding, selfless individual isn't a good thing, but mass communication is carefully set to manage the opinion of the populace within a narrow band of awareness and differing views.

Governments in democracies don't run the country. There are much more powerful groups that lie behind government. It is the interests of these supranational, supragovernmental organizations that you need to be careful of if you want to lose weight and feel great.

You need to start to be very careful who and what you listen to and start to see the wood for the trees.

Let's take a look at how it works.

Creating a smoke screen

The tobacco industry, for example, was clever. It managed to create the general perception that smoking was cool, sophisticated, street smart. The cigarette became an icon of sex, youth, vitality and freedom. And so people would be convinced to struggle through the initiation ritual – to cough and gag their way through their first cigarettes and, by the time they were 'cool', to be addicted to a drug that would make them feel terrible and eventually kill them.

Although the tobacco industry was successful at convincing men to smoke, it struggled with 'respectable' women. Middle-class women found it distasteful and uncouth to smoke. So the tobacco people staged a PR stunt that was probably the beginning of 'spin' as we know it.

A group of debutantes was organized to march publicly in New York. These 'sophisticated' young ladies each smoked a cigarette and held the burning sticks up as icons of freedom and independence for women.

The whole pre-arranged stunt was photographed and the pictures spread worldwide through the papers. Smoking was, virtually overnight, made respectable for women.

The role of tobacco in cancer began to emerge in the 1950s. This caused panic in the tobacco industry and a PR crisis management campaign was launched to protect the tobacco franchise...

Controlling the facts

An organization called the Tobacco Industry Research Committee (TIRC) was formed. This organization took full-page advertisements proclaiming that the tobacco industry would engage fully in the research process and cooperate with health officials. This was one way of lulling their existing and potential customers into a false sense of security.

The TIRC hired a leading cancer specialist to front the organization and to enhance its credibility. This organization trawled the literature for conflicting and inconclusive tobacco-related research and would produce papers for media release to confuse the issue. Meanwhile the tobacco industry doubled its advertising expenditure.

In the 1960s the TIRC was renamed and it became the Council for Tobacco Research (sounds more independent doesn't it?). This strategy – creating independent-sounding organizations as fronts for industry – has been copied many times; the 'Milk Marketing Boards', for example, became the 'National Dairy Councils'. The Council for Tobacco Research ran an army of PR people and lobbyists who are reported to have been solely concerned with delaying actions and misleading the public.

Another tactic used by the tobacco industry was to set up consumer front groups who would act as campaigners on behalf of the industry. So the National Smokers Alliance was formed (NSA). Front groups like this can be used as covers for research, the production of 'independent' reports and media spinning press releases and news items.

Of course the saga of tobacco is still unravelling. As small initiatives are made by government to protect consumers, we find that tobacco kills just as many people now as it did fifty years ago and that the tobacco industry is as profitable as it ever was. When one market closes down there is no compunction by the tobacco industry to run and take advantage of less well-regulated markets.

The same thing happens with pharmaceutical drugs and with food. Any evidence of negative side effects is dealt with in the same way using a series of public relations and lobbying tactics.

Imagine a global food manufacturer caught running a deadly scam selling infant formula to mothers in Third World countries. The company gives away 'free samples' of the product – just enough to stop the woman lactating so she is then bound to buy the product to feed her baby. These women live in poor, unhygienic conditions, often can't afford the formula and dilute it with contaminated water. This 'free formula' campaign causes misery, disease and deaths.

The resulting publicity leads to an international boycott of the company's products: infant formula, chocolate, instant coffee, canned products…

The company's response?

To set up a front organization. Perhaps call it the 'Coordination Centre for Nutrition' – an impressive, solid-sounding name. Use this organization to create a strategy to break the boycott. This front organization could set up a subsidiary headed by a former secretary of state or other high-up ex-official, professor or scientist – anyone who has public credibility and who is, more importantly, on the side of the rogue manufacturer.

The subsidiary organization might be called the 'Infant Formula Assessment Commission' (or some other credible and independent-sounding name). The advisory board of this group would entice members of the boycott groups to make them feel they were now participating in the solution. The boycotters would have to join. After all, if they didn't they would be choosing not to help and would be undermining their own position. If they did join, they would lend the group credibility – and undermine their own position. Either way, it's win-win to the killer infant formula company. Over time, the boycott loses its strength, the food company wins its war of attrition. The sorry saga is buried in history and few will remember – except, of course, for the Third World mothers who lost their children because a well-known food company cared more for profits than it did for health and well-being.

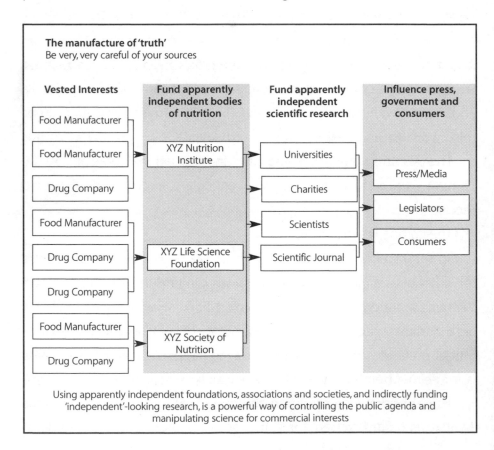

The manufacture of 'truth'
Be very, very careful of your sources

Using apparently independent foundations, associations and societies, and indirectly funding 'independent'-looking research, is a powerful way of controlling the public agenda and manipulating science for commercial interests

The setting-up of spurious front groups, illicit charities and scapegoat activist groups, and the creation of bogus experts, is a very effective strategy for misleading the media and government officials. The bigger and stronger you can make the front, and the more independent you can make it appear, the better.

Where's the evidence?

You don't have to look too hard for evidence of all this. Go onto the internet and type the words 'nutrition', 'diet', 'foundation', 'association' and 'organization' into a search engine. You will be confronted by a very long list of organizations. Which ones can you rely on and which can you not? Here's what to do:

Find a big respected, named organization in your country. Go to their website and take a look around. Then write to them as follows:

First letter: Request an annual report and audited accounts, and ask about any money received from commercial interests.

Second letter: Ask again. Keep asking until you hear back from them.

You will have varying degrees of success with different organizations. But the biggest and best-known names, when you dig deep enough, are frequently funded by food manufacturers who use these front organizations to further their corporate interests and lobby hard in favour of their current commercial freedoms: to market junk foods in limitless quantities, without warnings or meaningful labels, to consumers who are left in utter confusion by conflicting reports in newspapers and from different nutrition 'advisers'.

What went on, and is still going on with tobacco, is currently going on with food and nutrition. The upshot is that we live in an environment of nutritional chaos that is being deliberately orchestrated to confuse us as consumers and to hamstring the legislators.

WHO's right?

At the moment, the World Health Organization is working on new guidelines for maximum levels of food components that are damaging to health. These include refined sugar, saturated fat and excess salt; just three of a thousand 'food' components that are contributing to disease and death in our 'civilized' world. The sugar industry was reported as being furious at the WHO guidelines, which say that sugar should account for no more than ten per cent of a healthy diet. The sugar industry's response was that the WHO review, carried out by international experts, was 'scientifically flawed'. It was revealed that the sugar industry in the US threatened to bring the World Health Organization to its knees by demanding that Congress end its funding unless the WHO scrapped its guidelines on healthy eating. The sugar peddlers believe that a quarter of our food and drink intake can safely consist of sugar.

The Livetetic guideline is that no more than five per cent of any diet should consist of refined or processed sugar and there is absolutely no requirement for any refined sugar at all in an optimally healthy diet.

Manufacturers of refined and processed food are now in the spotlight.

Refined sugar is not a food. It is a chemical drug that causes damage even in small quantities. It is completely unnecessary in a healthy diet.

It is likely that the fight over refined and processed foods will be bigger, dirtier and uglier than the battle over tobacco. The tobacco scam is going to look like a kindergarten scrap compared with the blazing war that is about to unfold over

> *You can rest assured that where markets and profits are threatened there are very few scruples.*

'food'. The battle lines are drawn. There is a great deal at stake. The 'experts', lawyers and lobbyists are poised to defend the trade in junk sold as food.

Most scientific research is carried out by commercial interests. Many people think that a drug has to be proven safe and effective before it can be sold to the public. Well, that is the idea. But, in reality the game is to convince a government panel that the drug is safe and effective.

What's the difference between proof and convincing a panel that you have proof?

There is nothing to stop a drug manufacturer from running a series of research exercises with all the researchers bound by confidentiality and non-disclosure agreements. The research that is not positive can then be suppressed and ignored for the purposes of regulatory approval. The company can then go on to adjust methodology and/or terms of reference until, eventually, there is enough convincing data, and these will be the papers that are shown to the regulators.

Imagine you are a global agrochemical concern and you made a synthetic hormone that was designed to be injected into cattle to make them produce more milk. Imagine that this hormone, in late stages of testing, showed it had potentially devastating health consequences. What might you do, having invested some $500 million so far? Go back to the drawing board? Or might you be tempted to suppress the evidence, adjust the results and get it out to market as soon as possible?

We live in an environment where we cannot truly rely on science. Actually that isn't fair to science, for there are many dedicated, honest and thorough scientists who do great work. We live in an environment where we cannot rely on the use and the reporting of science.

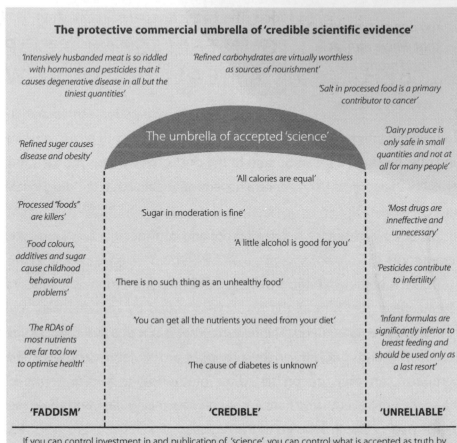

The protective commercial umbrella of 'credible scientific evidence'

'Intensively husbanded meat is so riddled with hormones and pesticides that it causes degenerative disease in all but the tiniest quantities'

'Refined carbohydrates are virtually worthless as sources of nourishment'

'Salt in processed food is a primary contributor to cancer'

The umbrella of accepted 'science'

'Refined suger causes disease and obesity'

'Dairy produce is only safe in small quantities and not at all for many people'

'All calories are equal'

'Processed "foods" are killers'

'Sugar in moderation is fine'

'Most drugs are inneffective and unnecessary'

'A little alcohol is good for you'

'Food colours, additives and sugar cause childhood behavioural problems'

'There is no such thing as an unhealthy food'

'Pesticides contribute to infertility'

'You can get all the nutrients you need from your diet'

'The RDAs of most nutrients are far too low to optimise health'

'Infant formulas are significantly inferior to breast feeding and should be used only as a last resort'

'The cause of diabetes is unknown'

'FADDISM' | **'CREDIBLE'** | **'UNRELIABLE'**

If you can control investment in and publication of 'science' you can control what is accepted as truth by experts. If most 'science' is directly or indirectly funded by industry and if the journals are selective in publication based on politics and commerce then 'science' will continue to be an unreliable source of 'truth'. So when expert groups review the published 'science' to find an answer it's like going to look for trees in a train tunnel. You need to get out of the tunnel to find out what is going on.

Science has been used consistently over the last 100 years to further commercial interests at the expense of truth. If we rely on the body of evidence that resides in peer-reviewed literature we will find that most of it has been funded directly or indirectly by commercial interests that have a particular angle on the subject in question.

And this is how you can end up with swathes of intelligent, honest, well-intentioned people who are convinced that junk is food.

I call the process… ignorruption.

IGNORRUPTION – THE ART OF MAKING INTELLIGENT PEOPLE BEHAVE IN A REALLY STUPID WAY

Ignorruption is the process by which otherwise intelligent and well-intentioned people are conned into believing and propagating distorted and potentially damaging beliefs about how things operate. If 80–90 per cent of peer-reviewed research is funded directly or indirectly by commercial interests, and those interests will only publish research that meets their requirements, then it is not difficult to see, when an 'independent' government review of the literature is undertaken, that it produces a result that confirms what the industry fronts and experts said all along.

This is one way in which ignorruption works. It is a way of keeping people in the dark. Get the general acceptance that the peer-reviewed literature is the only acceptable source of 'credible' science. Overwhelm the peer-review process with commercially funded research. Control the peer-review journals so that they only accept favourable papers. In this way you can 'control' science.

Ignorruption is insidious in our health services and in our nutritional institutions. It has been going on so long that we now have generations of nutrition 'experts' who believe the most idiotic scenarios and ideas. They dare not challenge the establishment because they, like Galileo with his 'ridiculous' round earth theory, will be condemned as heretics.

Monkey poles

I once heard a story about a social scientist who did an experiment with monkeys. He wanted to understand if and how they learned from one another. His experiment involved placing a monkey in a large, open cage.

> *'Ignorruption' is corruption of beliefs by ignorance*

There were various activities provided in the cage, and in the middle was a pole, at the top of which was a large bunch of fresh, ripe bananas.

One of the monkey's immediate actions was to see the bananas and start shinning up the pole. However, the scientist had rigged up a series of high-powered water sprays. When the monkey was one third of the way up, the spray jets were triggered and he was knocked off the pole by icy cold water. The monkey was tenacious; he tried again, only to be knocked down once more by the icy jets. And so it went on throughout his first day. He tried a dozen more times, each time becoming a little more wary and less committed. On the second day he tried once and, having been drenched yet again, he gave up.

On the third day the scientist introduced a second monkey. This monkey went for the pole straight away but the first monkey pulled him back and would not let him climb. Monkey 2 kept trying, but Monkey 1 eventually convinced him it wasn't a good idea and he didn't try again.

Next day a third monkey was introduced. Again, its immediate action was to head for the pole. This time Monkeys 1 and 2 pulled him away forcefully. They would not let him climb and their combined attempts encouraged the third monkey not to bother. But by now, the scientist had switched off the water jets.

On the next day the first monkey was taken out and a new monkey (Monkey 4) was introduced in his place. This monkey also went for the pole but was convinced by the remaining two not to try. What was interesting now was that none of those monkeys had experienced the water jets, but they wouldn't climb the pole to get a banana because they had been taught that it was a bad idea.

The scientist now had three monkeys in a cage and none of them would climb the pole to get a banana and none of them knew why! The monkeys were ignorrupts. They had their own and their peers' best interests at heart but their actions no longer had relevance. Their perception of reality was flawed and they were acting on a lie, or in this case, misinformation. It hadn't started out that way but they were ignorrupt just the same.

And so ignorruption is the most insidious of corruptions. It can convince the most intelligent of people to follow paths that are grotesquely misguided. Well-meaning, intelligent, well-intentioned people will follow wrong paths because they trust the people who teach them, and believe that the narrow bands of references to which they are exposed are indicative of the truth.

The territory of health and nutrition is riddled with ignorruption. Processed 'food' and pharmaceuticals are two of the largest and most profitable industries on earth. Virtually anything will be done to protect their franchise.

GM foods

Take for example the huff and puff about genetically modified food. One of the main ideas behind GM is that the company that acts quickly enough will be able to monopolize the market for crop seed and have farmers dependent on them for pesticides. The promise is for crops that deliver better yields, using less contaminants – but the reality is far from this, as experience with GM crops is showing quite the opposite; lower yields, contamination of surrounding organic crops and, in some cases, mutations in wildlife.

GM technology is about controlling markets and making money – the other ideas for it seem to have been put on the back burner for now.

We know very little about this unnecessary technology other than the fact that it is going through the ignorruption process.

The question remains – is GM food safe?

Genetically modified foods cannot be proved safe. At the very least they haven't been around long enough to see what the long-term impact will be. The commercial interests that promote them may convince the regulators to license their new products – but they will not necessarily be safe. The strategy of food and drug producers is to make money for as long as they can before science is able to prove any damaging effects. Fortunately for the food industry it is very difficult to scientifically prove connections between specific foods and any disease or deformity.

The pattern is well tested. We have heard the GM food issue compared with that of BSE. It seems a relevant 'food' example. But there are many more appropriate and spine-chilling analogies.

Thalidomide was a licensed drug that caused deformity in babies. Thousands of infants in 48 countries paid the price of their parents listening to the scientists who pronounced thalidomide 'safe'.

Thalidomide was vigorously defended by scientists until the day it was removed from use.

DES (diethylstilbestrol) was hailed as a wonder drug. It was given to millions of women before scientists connected it with causing cell cancers and deformities of the reproductive tract: not in the people who took it, but in their teenage daughters. It has since been implicated in deformities in the brain, the pituitary and the mammary glands of developing babies. Those children have paid the price of their mothers listening to the scientists who pronounced DES 'safe'.

PCBs (polychlorinated biphenyls) are a family of chemicals used in a myriad of industrial and consumer products. Over 50 years, 3.4 billion pounds of PCBs made their way into the environment. They entered the food chain, and now your body and every body on earth is contaminated with them. PCBs can be found in fat, hair and breast milk. Researchers have shown that animals polluted with minute quantities of PCBs can have suppressed immune systems, deformities of the uterus and Fallopian tubes, and suffer from failed pregnancies. Emerging evidence suggests that PCBs can cause brain damage to babies in the womb and they have been put forward as potential contributors to behavioural problems and breast cancer. It has been reported that in some areas the average European or American breastfeeding baby receives five times the allowable daily level of PCBs set by international health standards for a 150-pound adult.

PCBs were introduced in the late 1920s. For decades they were sold by one of the world's largest agrochemical concerns. This company defended their use for a long, long time, using any tactics they could to keep their poisonous compound on the market. Every human alive today is paying the price of the scientists who so strongly defended PCBs for 50 years. The agrochemical company that damaged your health with PCBs is now one of the major proponents of GM food. They have never paid damages or made reparations for the permanent pollution of the planet with this deadly concoction.

Thalidomide, DES and PCBs all owe their devastating potency to their hormone-like effects on the body. They are chemically similar to natural hormones and are capable of interfering with important bodily processes even in the most minute quantities. This connection was not made when they were pronounced 'safe'. Science made the connections later, after the profits had been made. Hundreds of other products remain on sale simply because the effects they have are less obvious or not so well studied.

What is the relevance of these non-food examples for genetically modified foods? Indeed, for any food grown unnaturally in artificially fertilized soil and using toxic compounds in order to control pests?

Drugs tend to have more potent effects on the body than food.

Even so, a drug will only be removed if there is a clear and obvious problem. Usually the scientists will fight for years before a drug or chemical is removed from sale.

Food producers tend to get away with potentially unsafe products for much longer. The adverse effects are more subtle and they are harder to prove. People die slowly from bad food. Food additives and processed food have the potential to harm people but usually in a way that is insidious. They are ignored because the effects are not obvious enough to embarrass a government minister. The food industry can literally get away with murder.

The line between drugs and chemicals and food is narrowing all the time. Commercial chemical, biochemical and food concerns ask us now to trust them with genetically modified food. Blindly, our appointed ministers in government listen and consider licensing these products. 'We are confident they are safe,' the regulators say. For they do not see any visible deformity, any direct connection, any short-term effect so disturbing that the public won't accept it.

What will it take?

Government ministers and legislators may say they are fully satisfied with the safety of genetically modified crops. It's a safe position for them to take. The chance of pinning disease or deformity on a specific food is highly unlikely; far less likely than a drug. This is a fact that the food industry trades upon again and again. The legislators speak in apparent ignorance of the issues. They are ignorrupts. Their paymasters in the agribusiness are happy and the legislators are unlikely to be proved wrong while they are in office. But that doesn't make them right.

Science cannot prove that genetically modified food is safe. It can, at best, suggest that with current knowledge the risks appear to be small.

Common sense says that messing with the very fabric of life, with the genetic order of things, is the ultimate stupidity. Whatever the outcome of the debate, we will not know until it is too late. As we have already seen, today 80 per cent of humans in the developed world will die, unnecessarily, from a degenerative disease such as heart disease, diabetes or cancer: diseases that virtually do not exist among those who do not eat refined and processed foods. Is it the sugar, salt, pesticides, colourings, additives, that are to blame? The answer is 'yes', all of them, but because the shallow, two-dimensional framework of 'science' doesn't like multiple causations or effects we continue to be allowed to buy foods contaminated with these pollutants. It is killing our children who are now obese, hyperactive, allergic, and predisposed to diabetes, heart disease and cancer. And that's before we even begin with the manipulation of genes.

When the planet is contaminated with unrecognizable mutant food, and our grandchildren are suffering with inexplicable new illnesses, will science then be able to make the connection? Probably not. Even if it does, there will be little that can be done.

One thing is certain, any physical or mental degeneration caused by the consumption of genetically modified food will create a ready market for a pharmaceutical industry that depends on disease for its profits.

It's a beautiful commercial cycle.

SELF-RELIANCE – TEST YOUR REFERENCES

So what is to be done? Self-reference is the solution. Rely on yourself. You're smart, you're able, you can work it out. Imagine if there was an easy way to lose weight that was obvious, did not involve deprivation and left you brighter, smarter, more energetic, sexier, more vital and enjoying a sense of total well-being, with a side benefit of freedom from degenerative disease.

You now know enough about how 'science' and 'news' can be manipulated to throw you off your beliefs, leaving you in a position where you accept that dangerous is safe and effective is ineffective.

Welcome to a new world. One where you are the boss; a world in which the way you feel is dictated by you alone. Where what happens around you does not impact on you directly but merely offers you an opportunity to reflect and to decide what to do about it.

Get yourself a glass of water. Any good drinking water will do. Still or sparkling – it doesn't matter. Even from the tap will be OK. Get the water before you read further and drink it.

Take a long deep breath before each sip. After you have breathed out sip the water and notice how it feels in your mouth. Swallow. Feel the water enter your body and how natural it feels. Notice the temperature change as it goes down your throat and enters your stomach. Breathe and sip again. Relax, sit up and feel the effect of the water as it goes down. If you soften your shoulders and relax your eyelids as you pull yourself up from the tip of your head by an imaginary thread, notice the water leave your stomach and enter your bloodstream.

Sip the water again and notice the feeling in your toes. Breathe. Sip. Swallow. That water is totally natural in your body. About 70 per cent of your body is water. If you were a single-celled balloon and you were punctured so the water flowed out, you would reduce to about a quarter of your size.

But you are not. You are made up of about 75 trillion tiny cells. All of them contain water. All of them need water. Water acts as a way of moving things around. The fluidity that bathes your cells depends on the purity of the water you take in. The ability of your cells to stay fresh and hydrated depends on your water intake.

Breathe deeply. Sip from your water. Notice it reach your cells. No digestion required.

Sip, swallow, throat, stomach, bloodstream, cells. In a heartbeat.

> *We cannot stay the same. With every action we choose either to regenerate or degenerate.*

That drink of water will change your destiny; such a simple thing to do but even simpler not to do! Finish your glass of water and continue. The way your mind works, your ability to receive messages, your capacity for independent thought and concentration depend on having enough water in your system.

Spend five minutes just noticing your body. Feel every breath. Feel the water you have just drunk moving around your system. Imagine it moving in and around your cells. Feel refreshed.

Staying the same isn't an option for any of us. With every breath, every sip, every mouthful, every thought and every movement we influence our destiny. We are responsible for our well-being. For most who read this book there is no one forcing them to eat or drink anything. Everything goes in by choice.

We alone choose how we feel, how we look and how well we are.

Welcome to Livetetics.

MOTIVATION – WHY WE DO WHAT WE DO

D id you actually drink that glass of water and pause to listen to your body? If you did then you are to be congratulated. You are already well on your way to your perfect destiny.

Many people don't bother – think they will do it later – just want to get on. 'I get the point without doing it'. Go back and do it. If you do, you succeed. If you don't, you don't succeed. The choice is complete success or less complete success: your destiny is yours. Get the glass of water, turn back the page and do it! Action is the grand thing.

So why is it that we choose to do some things and not others? What is our motivation?

There are two primary motivating factors. The first is pleasure. The second is pain. They come in that order. First we are moved to obtain pleasure. Second we are moved to avoid pain.

And so we find pleasurable things easy to do. We find activities that are pleasurable, foods that are pleasurable and places that are pleasurable. Pleasure is a craving for most of us.

But, if there is pain involved we will take evasive action. Most people will not deliberately drink a cocktail of arsenic and battery acid. The almost instantaneous rupture of their throat, the internal bleeding and rapid, painful death make this something that is best avoided. But people will smoke cigarettes that deliver a massively increased chance of a painful and premature death. Why does this happen?

We have already discussed how smokers have been deceived by the chemistry of smoking into thinking that it is pleasurable. Smokers smoke because the drugs they inhale make them feel better than when they are not smoking. But they only need the drug because the smoking is making them feel bad. Create a product that makes people sick and make it so that they crave it because they think it makes them feel better. Then create an environment in which they are fooled into thinking the addiction is much more powerful than it really is – so they are conditioned to find it difficult to give up.

It's brilliant, isn't it?

Stealth harms health

It is also true that the prospect of pain is easily ignored if the incremental effect is not noticeable. And so we find that the avoidance of disease is not a great motivator. The smoker knows he is killing himself but the pain of death from suffocation and excruciating lung pain is a long way off – for now the pleasure seems worth it. So the next cigarette is lit up and sucked on. A large part of the brand positioning of smoking is that of freedom and independence and devil-may-care, so many smokers believe that sucking the smoke from burning leaves makes them look daring and brave. The 'pleasure' exceeds the pain and the decision is made.

However, if you can bring the pain forward, then people often find it easier to give up smoking. Someone who is diagnosed with lung cancer or who gets a condition where the smoke itself causes pain often then finds it rather straightforward to give up.

Expectant mothers, too, now know enough about the risks to their unborn babies and find the prospect of a damaged child enough of an inducement to give up smoking instantly – even if they have tried and not succeeded many times before.

This is natural. If you were to drop a frog into a pan of scalding water it would jump out immediately. But if the frog was allowed to swim in a pan of water that is gradually heated, it is likely to

> *We are driven first by pleasure and then by pain*

stay swimming until it is too late, and be killed by the temperature of the water.

Let's take our battery acid and arsenic example. You wouldn't touch it would you? Unlikely. But what if it were chemically altered so that the burning of your throat was less noticeable, imperceptible even. What if it were altered so that the arsenic didn't act so fast? Then perhaps add some gorgeous, comforting ingredients and serve it warm and frothy in lovely places. Show pictures of people, fashionable people, enjoying the cocktail in a happy, social environment. The people are 'cool', they are having fun, they are enjoying life, they are free. Someone offers you a sip, it tastes great. You want some of that life. Everybody's doing it, which means it must be OK.

You go for it. You go to the shop that sells it. The shop smells wonderful. The décor is trendy. Other people are in there drinking the liberating, cool, fashionable, great tasting liquid. You order. You're in. The drink tastes great, it gives you a buzz, you don't drop dead. 'Hmm', you think, 'I like this, this is me – I'm part of this. I'll do this again'.

The craving for pleasure is immense. And we find many ways to get it. One way is from putting things in our mouths, chewing and swallowing them. In fact, for the most part, we now eat and drink for pleasure. We know that many so-called 'foods' are not good for health but we continue to eat them just the same. We use 'food' as a drug, for pleasure.

The fact that drinking alcohol or coffee, for example, has a negative impact on health makes no difference to most. When beer or wine is sipped, the mind is not focused on the deterioration of liver function, the erosion of the nervous system, the poisoning of body cells or the increased risk from degenerative disease. After a glass or two, the pleasure is all that matters. When coffee is taken, its effect on the nervous system is not considered; the stress on the liver is not foremost in our minds.

The imbalances coffee creates in blood sugar and the fact that it encourages the deposition of fat on our organs and bodies is not what we think about; we do not think for a moment about how it stops us effectively digesting essential minerals, nor the damage it can cause to an unborn child or to the reproductive capacity of a young woman or man.

Sharing coffee and alcohol with friends is an institution. It is a pleasant, comforting, relaxing and refreshing thing to do. Or that's how we have been conditioned to feel about it. It's the same with cake, biscuits and snacks of a thousand varieties. We eat them for pleasure. We eat them because we think they make us feel better.

Evolution has a lot to do with this preoccupation with pleasure and food. We have some evolutionary tastes that have been set up to help us make good food choices.

We crave sugar.

We crave fat.

We crave salt.

In the natural world, however, all of these food components are either rare or they come in forms that are nutritionally rich.

SUGAR

In the natural world sweet foods are fruits and berries and root vegetables. These foods are rich sources of living nutrients and nourishment.

FAT

Natural, essential fats come from oily fish and fresh raw nuts and seeds.

These essential fats are critical for the growth and functioning of our brains and the operation of a thousand different body functions. We need these essential fats in very tiny quantities. Our natural requirement for fat is less than a spoon a day.

SALT

Salt contains an important mineral called sodium that forms charged particles known as ions. Sodium ions, along with chloride and potassium ions, are needed to keep equilibrium between the inside and outside of our cells. Sodium is scarce on land in the natural world. We have a taste for it and our bodies are designed to hang on to it – but too much can be very harmful.

These primeval cravings are designed to be helpful and drive us to sensible food choices, but Western mankind's access to these food components has changed dramatically. Now we have access to sweet 'foods' that have no nutritional value at all. Our food is liberally laden with all manner of fats; manufactured and mutated fats that our bodies find hard to tell apart from the good fats, and contains very few of the essential fats we evolved to crave. Salt is liberally added to foods so that we will like the taste of them and so, of course, keep buying them.

And so our evolutionary pleasure senses are used against us. The manufactured 'foods' that are designed to appeal to our cravings are, just like the cigarette, giving us an illusion of well-being when in fact they create long-term pain. Sweet, salty and fatty foods can be addictive. People find it very difficult to reduce or eliminate them from their intake: their consumption can create hormonal and metabolic shifts that set up cravings and the suppression of our natural ability to know when we've had enough.

The result of eating these redundant foods is shrouded in confusion and 'scientific' conflict. We already know why: because manufacturers have little interest in warning you about their deadly effects or encouraging you to limit your consumption. But common sense can save the average person from being baffled by the corporate messages that try to convince us these products should be classed as foods, and sold to us as though they have nutritional value. There is good news, however. Livetetics isn't going to ask you to give anything up that you don't want to; instead it will ask you to gain things that you do.

Back to our motivations.

The ultimate pleasure is to achieve a goal that is compelling. You may remember that we started the process of describing our perfect day a while back. It is now time to develop that goal. Turn back to page 43 and look at what you wrote down about that perfect day, your perfect life.

Visualize how you want to be.

Sit for a few moments and really create a vision of how it is going to be.

Stand up. Come on, stand up. (It's OK to feel strange about standing up in response to words on a page!)

Stand the way you will stand when you feel totally full of energy. It will help if you relax your shoulders and lift your head gently so that you are looking straight ahead. Feel as though there is a fine thread tugging at the top of your head, lifting it upwards. From the top of your neck feel a stretch that goes all the way down to the base of your spine.

Breathe.

Starting with your toes squeeze and relax the muscles in your feet, your calves, your thighs, your buttocks, your stomach, your back, your chest, your shoulders, your fingers, your forearms, your upper arms, your face – there are lots of muscles in your face. And you will have to make some really weird faces to stretch and relax them all (my apologies if you are in a train!).

Having done this, stand as perfectly balanced as you can and feel the way you are going to feel when you have achieved perfection. Stay as yourself and go into a dream where you can see yourself the way you want to be – as you. If you don't find this easy to do, then make a picture of yourself the way you are going to be. Notice how you will breathe. Hear what you will hear. See what you will see. Notice how this new you looks and feels.

Walk around yourself in your mind – look closely at your body the way it is going to be, notice how it feels to be in that new body. Notice how you breathe and how breathing makes you feel. Notice how you can relax the little muscles at the side of your mouth and, as you do, notice the feeling inside that you get from beginning the process of change. Step into a new you. Try the new you on like a set of new clothes. Shuffle in so you feel comfortable.

Inside you, right now, is your perfect body and, a heartbeat away, are all the feelings of euphoria and ecstasy that you deserve.

Make this picture regularly. Talk to yourself about how it is going to be. Be gentle on yourself; remember you've got where you are today by doing the best you could. Your decisions were always intended to have beneficial effects. If you've made a few mistakes then that's fine. They can be corrected. It is never too late to change easily and quickly.

It's going to be a blast, this Livetetic process.

There are no calories to count.

You can eat freely.

You will learn to take responsibility for your decisions.

You will never go on a diet again.

You will feel far more self-sufficient and in control.

It is all about reclaiming pleasure and contentment.

So what have we learned?

BELIEFS

Our beliefs are all important. What we believe to be true, what we believe about food, what we believe about our personal capabilities is what drives our actions. And our actions drive our destiny. How we feel, how we behave, how we look are the foundation of what we will become.

CHANGE

We are changing. Like it or not, with every breath, with every sip, with every bite, with every movement. We are either regenerating or degenerating. Our bodies are in a state of constant flux and interchange with the environment. Our actions determine the direction of the change. Our beliefs and feelings drive our actions. We will change whatever we do. WE can decide what we will change into.

REFERENCES

Internal references are more important and solid than external references. We cannot necessarily rely on commonly held wisdom for the truth. It is important to focus on our internal references, using our internal feelings rather than taking external cues. Self-reference is the most powerful force for positive change. It delivers independence, control and freedom.

SCIENCE

'Science' does not necessarily deliver the truth. 'Science' is a tool used most often to guide people into believing certain things. The greater part of 'science' is paid for by companies that want to sell products and steer government and legislation in certain directions. Be very wary of media reports about 'science' – look rather for results and model your beliefs upon those who appear to get them.

EXPERTS

Sometimes the 'experts' can't see the wood for the trees. How can two scientists spend their entire lives in diligent, intelligent and honest pursuit of the truth only to come up with completely opposing points of view? Integrity and intelligence does not guarantee truth. Be a child. Challenge the dogma and ask the dumb questions. The dumb questions are often the most powerful.

IGNORRUPTION

Remember the monkey pole. Three monkeys that would not climb the pole to get a fresh banana and none of them knew why. Out-of-date beliefs and 'common wisdom', no matter how well-intentioned, can hamstring people into idiotic and destructive behaviour. Look around for your monkey poles and challenge your beliefs.

MOTIVATION

We are driven by pleasure and pain. No one does anything that they do not believe has a positive outcome. Obtaining pleasure is our primary motivation, followed by the avoidance of pain. To make change we must have a compelling goal, a compelling future that makes the change pleasurable. We should also understand what is going on!

You now have a clear vision of what you want to achieve. Feeling fantastic, looking fantastic and being healthy, vital and totally well in every way. The way you were designed to be!

Your body, working with you

Your body, working with you

When you buy a car or a piece of electrical equipment, you get an owner's manual, a handbook that gives you information about looking after your new possession. It tells you how to make sure you get the best performance and the longest life out of your acquisition. It has information on how to work the controls and how to use it safely and effectively.

Before you are allowed to take a motorized vehicle on a public highway you have to demonstrate that you are competent to drive it. You have to show that you know the rules and are able to perform a series of essential manoeuvres. There are signs you need to understand and skills you need to demonstrate you have. This is all for your safety and for the safety of others.

The rules are clear, they are well defined and they are explicit. There is very little room for interpretation and misunderstanding. At a red light you stop. Not sometimes, always! It isn't OK to jump red lights 'in moderation'. A little stop-light risk isn't good for you!

When it comes to putting oil in your engine, the type of oil and its grade is clearly spelled out. It is not OK to throw in any old oil; try using hair oil instead of engine oil and you're in trouble. The same with water. You need to keep your engine's cooling system clean and topped up. It is not OK to fill it with cola. It just doesn't work!

With your body, you are on your own. Nobody tells you how it works – not in any really useful way. You just have to guess. You pick things up as you go along. Like learning to speak. You copy those around you, you listen to your parents, you watch your peers and friends and you do things that fit in with them. You watch television, you read books, you listen to your teachers. All of these people, family, friends and a variety of celebrities act as role models for you.

The trouble is that three quarters of your role models are dying of unnecessary degenerative diseases. They die fat, unhealthy and with incorrect opinions and attitudes.

Trying to find out how best to operate your body and mind can be very confusing. Your parents might encourage you to eat fresh fruit and vegetables and discourage your consumption of sweets, soda and salty snacks. Yet they will shower you with chocolate and sweets and soda and crisps and biscuits on your birthday; a day that is a celebration of your life and your importance in their hearts.

If you are deprived of the junk foods that are everywhere around you, you will feel you are missing out. After all, a little of what you fancy won't do you any harm – will it? They wouldn't sell it to children if it hurt them – would they? Deliberately avoiding all of the 'treats' that everyone else is eating is seen to be 'faddy', 'on a diet', 'being good'. For children, choosing fruit instead of chocolate pudding is not a 'cool' option. Choosing salad rather than chips (over which salt is poured), is just not streetwise.

The teacher who holds up the colourful chart and tells our children, 'two portions from the meat, eggs and fish group, two portions from the dairy group' believes this to be good advice. My son showed me a science test paper in which he was expected to tick a box confirming that the statement, 'cakes are mainly made of starch and sugar which gives you lots of energy', was true. This is, once again, utterly misleading.

It starts at school

Ignorruption has thoroughly permeated our channels of education. Teachers are used as advertisements for 'foods' that have no place in the intake of a healthy child. Teaching materials are sometimes supplied by institutions created to sell meat, fish, eggs, sugar, milk and butter. The agricultural and food industry salesmen know: 'get them young and you get them for life'. Think about this next time you walk past the vending machine in the school lobby and the shiny cardboard collecting bins placed there by the well-meaning Parent-Teachers Association, so that children can be encouraged to eat crisps and chocolate and then save tokens from the wrappers, and so trade their health and bodies for new books and sports equipment.

To a certain extent, we have a latent belief that it is all natural and inevitable. We eat because we need to for survival. All foods are OK in moderation. We should eat from a wide variety of foods and take some exercise. Other than that, it's in the lap of the gods. If we get sick we go to the doctor to find out what is wrong and have it repaired, if possible. There isn't really much else to be done, is there? We know we should eat more fruit and vegetables, cut back on alcohol and avoid smoking but, other than that, we are what we are – aren't we? It's in our genes – isn't it?

These attitudes are very ineffective beliefs upon which to build an effective life. You are a winner. It is time to live like a winner. You have a perfect, incredible body that is designed to feel and look fabulous.

A winner? What do I mean?

Well, one of the things I know about you is that you won a very important race. It was a long time ago and you probably don't remember it. But you won it just the same.

To be conceived you had to win an amazing race. You beat hundreds of millions of other potential people to fertilize an egg and start your life. How does it feel to be the best of about 400,000,000 people?

Imagine yourself, standing in a crowd of people 5-10 times bigger than the entire population of the United Kingdom. You wait for the starting pistol and you're off. All of you in a massive crowd running – your life depending on it – to win the prize. And you win.

That's quite an achievement. Congratulations.

Educate yourself

But now you find yourself in your incredible body. What do you do next? The advice around you is all so confusing. One day we hear that taking food supplements can protect us from diseases. The next day we hear that they are unnecessary and cause diseases. Research from the supplement people one day, research from the drug people the next. All the news has an angle.

Whom should you believe?

You already know the answer. Believe no one except yourself. Read your owner's manual. What do you mean, you haven't got one? You're in charge of one of the most incredible, delicate, powerful, self-repairing, self-regulating, technologically complex machines on the planet and you don't have any clear instructions on how to use it?

Don't be ridiculous.

It's time to learn a little about yourself that you may not know. You've got the body, it came free with your life. It is an extraordinary machine. One day in the life of your body is enough to steal all the wonder from fiction. You are utterly incredible.

THE BODY WE DESERVE – HOW SHOULD IT BE?

We are living miracles. As you read this sentence, your heart, without you having to think about it, pumps blood around your body. That blood is pumped through about 60,000 miles of blood vessels. Blood carries fuel and nutrients to the 75 trillion cells in your body. 75 trillion! Each cell is an individual entity with its own set of tasks and functions, energy production plant, and capability to take in what it needs and send out what it doesn't. It also has the ability to reproduce itself in some cases. Your cells offload their waste and the rubbish is carried away by blood and lymph system, which transports it around until it can be eliminated.

If you heard a loud bang now that really scared you, your brain would trigger the release of a hormone that would immediately prepare you to deal with an emergency. Hormones are little chemical messengers that tell certain parts of your body to do certain things. They can reach just about any part in nano-seconds. You have an automatic 'fight or flight' reflex that prepares your entire body when you are frightened or shocked. You know what it's like – a scary noise or a near-miss in the car – there is a thud in your chest and your heart races, you breathe more deeply, your muscles are flexed, there is more sugar in your blood – you are ready. This is all because of the automatic release of a chemical messenger in one part of your body, which reaches all the other necessary parts before you can draw your next breath.

Your 9–12 pints of blood make about 4,000 trips a day around your body. In places the blood vessels are so tiny that they only let through one cell at a time. Your body has an internal transportation network that makes the road and rail network of this country look like a child's play mat or colouring book by comparison. Your skin contains about four million pores that give off moisture and help keep your body in balance. Skin is the largest organ of the body.

This is all coordinated by your brain without you having to think about it. Your liver uses about fifty primary different enzymes and a range of nutrients to detoxify and neutralize toxic substances that get into your blood and lymphatic systems, either from the outside or from the process of digesting your food and using nutrients for energy.

All of this happens without you having to do a thing.

Just notice your toes for a moment. Which of your feet is warmer? Notice how you can feel the blood flowing through your feet. If you really relax and pay attention you will notice that blood pulses through your feet in time with the rhythm of your heart. One moment the blood is in your heart, then it is in your feet.

At their best, our bodies are designed to be:

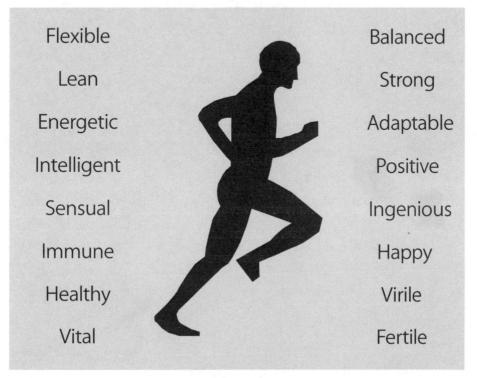

Flexible	Balanced
Lean	Strong
Energetic	Adaptable
Intelligent	Positive
Sensual	Ingenious
Immune	Happy
Healthy	Virile
Vital	Fertile

Your body is perfect. You are perfect. All the complicated, difficult things are taken care of. You are free to get on with living while your body takes care of its own perfect self. Just give it what it needs and it will look after you until the day you die – peacefully and in good health. In the meantime, you have the opportunity to live in a state of total vitality, total harmony, total well-being.

Your body is designed to be lean, strong and resilient. It fights off intruders, repairs itself when it is damaged, grows and replaces itself automatically over time. It is absolutely incredible.

If you believe anything less than this you are settling for second best and it is a sure sign that you have some beliefs and behaviours to adjust.

But to continue. You may have heard the expression, 'You are what you eat'. This isn't true. And this is where the story begins.

DIGESTION – WE ARE NOT WHAT WE EAT

The health of your digestive system is perhaps one of the most important influences on how good you feel and how great you look. Your digestive system is a wonder.

Your tube system

Have you ever thought of yourself as a tube? Well you are. Running through the middle of your body is a tube that is open, at either end, to the outside. It starts with your mouth and ends up at your anus. This tube is the central part of your digestive system. You get things into the tube by putting them in your mouth and swallowing. As they pass through you, your body has an opportunity to take useful nutrients from whatever you have put into it and then to dispose of the waste as solids, liquids and sometimes gas.

What happens in-between is very important. The process of digestion cannot be taken for granted. There are some things you must do for it to work well and you need to look after it. If it works well you can absorb what you need from your food. It will feed your body, help you feel full of energy and emotionally balanced, and make you lean and strong with great skin. However, if you don't pay attention to your digestion it can set up the conditions for food cravings, allergies, bad skin, depression, chronic energy deficiencies and immune problems.

Let's begin with looking at how your digestive tube deals with food.

TUBE STOP 1 – MOUTH

It all begins in your mouth. Chewing is the first phase of digestion. Your mouth produces saliva and this fluid begins the digestive process.

Just for amusement, go to a pizza restaurant. Go in and spend half an hour just watching the people as they eat.

Count how many times, on average, they chew their mouthfuls. Some people will shock you. They will tear off great chunks of pizza, gulp them down with barely a chew and then wash the rest down with a drink. If you have a good day you might see someone chew 5-10 times. It is unlikely that you will see anyone chew more than ten, maybe 15, times. We have not been taught to chew. We have forgotten how to chew.

> *Drink your food and chew your drink*

So why is it so important? Well, chewing breaks food down into small pieces. The smaller the pieces the more your digestive fluids can surround them. The more the fluids and enzymes can surround them the more easily they can be digested. Digestion actually starts in your mouth with important enzymes in your saliva getting the process going. If food does not stay in your mouth long enough, then digestion gets off to a false start.

My experience as a practitioner is that about 50 per cent of indigestion problems can be solved by teaching people to chew. Do not expect this news from the people that advertise antacids. It is much better for them that 'indigestion' be considered a medical disorder for which a chemical can be prescribed. No one ever made any money out of teaching people to chew. Incidentally, chewing can dramatically accelerate weight loss as the food is in your mouth for longer and so triggers the 'full' feeling sooner.

Go and get yourself an apple. Do it now.

Have you got it? Can't find one? Then get any piece of fruit. Haven't got a piece of fruit nearby? If you have no fruit nearby then you are going to get serious benefits from Livetetics! Get some fruit. Do it now.

Take a bite of your apple and chew it 50 times. Count the chews. As you chew you will notice how your reflex swallowing action takes liquid down into your body. Your tongue naturally keeps the remaining solids in your mouth and you can keep on chewing. Most people have to make a conscious effort not to swallow the mouthful before the 50 chews are up. By that time there is virtually nothing left to swallow. Well done, you just learned to 'drink your food'. This skill will help you lose weight, get better skin, feel more energetic, reduce your appetite, give you more nutrients to fuel your immune system and help ensure you get the most you can from your digestive system.

Practise chewing with the rest of your apple. Notice how the fruit freshens your mouth. Pay attention to it going down as you did with the water a little while ago. You will be able, if you really pay attention, to notice places in your body where you can actually feel the fruit nutrients working. It may be gentle warmth in certain places or a comfortable, slightly tingling feeling. These little feelings are your body using natural fuel to feed and nourish your cells.

We are learning, in this section, to use our digestion to convert food into positive energy and strength. If food is gulped and only partially broken down it has the potential to be converted into wasteful fat, toxic compounds and negative energy.

We have already talked about the exchange of atoms in our breathing. Eating is another, vital, exchange with our environment. The reason we eat is to extract energy and intelligence from food, then to assimilate that energy and intelligence into our bodies. The amount of energy and intelligence in different foods governs how much use it is to us.

Living, whole foods contain living energy and natural intelligence. Processed and refined foods generally contain lifeless substances.

The notion, for example, that refined sugar gives us energy requires a very blinkered view of nutrition – it is a commonly held view but it is not true. The sugar contains calories but these are an illusion of nutrition. We'll talk about this later (see page 139), but suffice it to say that your body will much better regulate food intake and hunger if you eat real food rather than manufactured imitations.

The thoroughness with which you chew your food is a decision you make every time you eat that will alter your path and determine your destiny. Livetetics is not about one great change or a major shift in behaviour or beliefs. It is about a myriad of tiny adjustments that have profound and powerful effects. Chewing? Can it really be this simple? Could you commit to chewing your food? You must, if you want a change in how you feel and look.

TUBE STOP 2 – STOMACH

Next stop on the tube is the stomach. This is where some other enzymes get involved; enzymes that operate alongside stomach acid to break down your well-chewed, liquefied food molecules into even smaller components. The acid is an important part of this process. Your stomach produces very strong acid – it would burn you if you stuck your finger in it – but the stomach wall is protected. The set-up of these enzymes and the acid production is triggered by the chewing process and your initial swallows. Production of adequate acid is dependent on there being enough water in your body, and also highly dependent on the presence of an important mineral called zinc. Fresh, raw fruit and vegetables are the best way to set up your digestive system.

Between chewing properly, drinking enough water and getting enough zinc you can permanently solve the majority of indigestion and acid reflux problems without needing any medication whatever. If you know someone who needs this information, please tell them.

This is not advice that is commonly given by doctors or pharmacists.

While we are talking about the stomach, it is worth noting that the digestive processes work best when it is partially empty. Now is a good time to make a connection between feelings of hunger and putting food in your mouth.

For the most part, we are not in tune with our hunger and satisfaction meters. The body has many very intricate instruments that measure body functions and set controls. These include temperature, the amount of sugar in your blood, the acidity of your body, the density of your bones, ionic balance and many others. Along with these measures are triggers that encourage you to eat when you need to take on more energy and to stop eating when you have had enough.

Modern foods and the way we live have interfered with these measures so that we do not know when we are hungry or when we have eaten enough. We are out of touch with the foods that make us feel vibrant and well and too frequently go for those that make us lethargic, depressed and fat. Food is now contaminated with a host of unnatural flavours, colours, preservatives, pesticides, refined sugar, excess salt, unnatural fats and a myriad of additives to help it flow, congeal, emulsify or generally behave in the way the manufacturer wants it to.

It is crucial to get back in touch with our natural, or 'real' appetite. We have been so bombarded with messages telling us what we should like to eat that getting back in touch with reality can be difficult. We often eat because we want a break, need something to do, we're with friends and it is a social thing to do, we crave some 'energy', we smell something appealing and want it; these are all reasons for eating that have nothing to do with our appetite or hunger.

A fundamental law of Livetetics is:

Eat when you are hungry
When you are not hungry – don't eat

So how do we know when we are hungry? Well, the hunger mechanism is there in all of us and it will be there for you if you let it emerge.

Some people feel hunger in their belly, some in their chest, some in their throat, some even in their legs. It doesn't matter where you feel it. The first trick is not to interrupt the process by eating before you feel hungry. If you wait, you will get your personal signal and know that it is time to eat. Revel in the feeling – it's probably the first time you've experienced it for quite a while!

It is likely that you are not used to recognizing your hunger. Fear not – there are lots of reasons. It might be that you eat before you feel hungry. You eat because it is break-time and eating is what is done during a break. You eat because your companions are eating. You eat because you are happy or as a celebration. You eat because it's lunchtime and lunchtime is a time to eat. You eat because the children didn't and it's a shame to waste it. You eat because you are bored. You eat because you are lonely. You eat because you feel fat and hopeless.

You can find a thousand reasons to eat, and none of them to do with your natural hunger to take on a little more energy and intelligence from your environment.

Some people have a fear of feeling hungry. The sensation of hunger scares them and they eat in advance of it to try and avoid it or ignore it. Why might this happen? Often it comes from childhood; being forced to clear a plate whether we wanted to or not; sensing a teacher's or a parent's disapproval if we said we weren't hungry; feeling we had to eat at a shared family meal. Such fear can come from all sorts of places and often people aren't consciously aware of it.

Hunger is a very natural and important sensation. It is a very pleasurable sensation. To feel genuinely hungry feels fabulous. We should enjoy this sensation more.

Let's have a go at getting back in touch with real, positive hunger. To begin with, you can get back in touch with it by using an imaginary scale:

Level	How you feel	What to do
Empty	Your stomach is uncomfortably empty. You are desperate to eat.	Don't get to this point – it is important to eat before you reach this level.
1	Your stomach is completely empty and you cannot feel the presence of any food from a previous meal. There is a sensation of hunger.	This is the point at which to start eating. Always begin with a glass of water and some fresh, raw food – fruit or salad.
2	You have the good feeling that you are eating slowly and comfortably. Or the feeling just after you have eaten and are comfortably digesting the food.	You do not feel hunger at this level. Eat well and slowly if you are enjoying a meal. Enjoy the process of digestion if you are between meals.
3	As you are eating you start to feel satisfied.	Pay attention to your food. Chewing, enjoying. Start to notice impending satisfaction.
4	The point of optimum comfort. You feel satisfied – there is no hunger nor discomfort.	Stop eating. (Even if there is food on your plate and another course on the menu!)
5	You have gone further than is comfortable. You begin to feel your abdomen swell a little, there is a latent heaviness.	Stop eating. Go for a gentle stroll and breathe deeply. Lie down for ten minutes and reflect on what made you eat too much. Look forward to stopping sooner next time.
Full	You can't eat another bite. Your stomach is full to the point of bursting – it is distended and uncomfortable.	Rest. Lie down and breathe deeply. Sleep if you can. Walk for an hour, breathe deeply, increase your pace. Commit to stopping at level 4 next time.

At the beginning, while getting back into the rhythm of your natural hunger, make a mental note of your satisfaction level before you eat anything. Write it down if you like: satisfaction level before – satisfaction level after. Eat at level 1 and stop eating at level 4.

We often eat to solve hungers other than those for food. Eating to solve loneliness will not do the trick. Eating because we are sad or angry won't make us happy or gentle. Eating because we feel lost will take us deeper into the woods. If we are moved to eat when we are not hungry for food then we must face what it is we are really hungry for.

If you find yourself about to eat when you are not hungry – stop for a moment. Ask yourself what you are actually hungry for. If you cannot answer the question, it doesn't matter. Just chuckle to yourself and be pleased that not eating when you might have done will take you closer to the solution. If you have the time and space, do something else rather than eat. Here are just a very few suggestions of what you might do:

- Have a bath

- Curl up in a comfortable chair and read a book

- Go for a walk and watch people – really watch them

- Phone a friend

- Write some sentences about what you really want

- Write a poem

- Do something for someone else

- Stand in an open space and breathe deeply – notice how every breath makes you feel better.

Food and feelings are very close together. We associate food with feelings. It is, after all, energy and intelligence we naturally want when we eat. But it is all mixed up these days. The manufacturers of food advertise so that we associate feelings with food. And so we are led to believe that chocolate is delicious and comforting and warming; that instant coffee is refreshing, enlivening, relaxing, even that it has something to do with relationships; that crisps are irresistible; that biscuits are sociable and chocolates a demonstration of thanks and gratitude. We are sold packages of feelings attached to sticks of fat and sugar and salt. Advertisements tell our children that sugared cereals are exciting and that sweets are sociable and fun. Crisps obtain attributes of success and coolness by being associated with celebrities and sports icons.

It is a confidence trick. Subconsciously we do realise this. It is making us sick and fat.

But with Livetetics you are in control. You can watch the TV advertisements and notice how the manufacturer of a packaged 'food' product doesn't sell you nutrition or energy or intelligence. He tries to sell you a bundle of feelings with it: 'be a good mother', 'obtain pleasure you can't measure', 'success', 'love'. And he sells you a concoction that is designed to trick you into believing it tastes good by exploiting your evolutionary, natural tastes for sugar and fat and salt. He then goes further by adding chemical flavours and sweeteners. Now the food manufacturers have worked out that people are beginning to see through this façade of feelings and that consumers actually want vitality, well-being and health. And so you start to see the words 'perfectly balanced', 'fresh', 'natural', 'rich in Vitamin C' appear on the labels. Advertisements show lithe people with glowing skin frolicking in fields with happy children and then the final picture of a cardboard box, a foil wrapper or a tin containing the latest product of the manufacturing and chemical plants.

Back to the stomach. It is important to know that processed sugar can slow down the secretion of gastric juices and inhibits the stomach's natural ability to move. When taken alone, sugars pass quickly from the stomach to the intestine. But when eaten in combination with other foods, refined sugar hangs around and can start an acid fermentation that fouls up the digestive process.

> *Get in touch with your natural hunger. Only eat when you are at level one. Stop when you are at level four. Notice every mouthful. Chew it well.*

Don't worry about the junk 'food' manufacturers. Livetetics will deliver you all the skills you need to see through their sales talk and misinformation and make better decisions about how to nourish your cells. Getting in touch with your digestion is a powerful step in the direction of freedom from junk sold as 'food'.

TUBE STOP 3 – INTESTINE

And so the journey continues. From the stomach into the intestine, a tube that winds into your body away from your stomach. In this tube, further breakdown, and digestion, take place. The intestinal tube has a surface that is made up of little finger-like protrusions, called villi, that significantly expand its surface area potential for absorption. In fact, if you spread out the surface of your intestine it would be about the size of a tennis court. These finger-like protrusions allow the food you are digesting to come into contact with the intestinal wall and facilitate the absorption of nutrients into tiny blood vessels, which then take the extracted energy and intelligence to parts of your body that need them.

This part of the digestive process needs looking after. There are a number of things that can mess up the absorption of nutrients.

Watch out for wheat bran. A lot of people eat this because they think it provides useful 'roughage' or fibre. In fact, wheat bran binds with zinc and calcium and inhibits their absorption. Wheat bran is also very rough. It can irritate the lining of the small intestine and interfere with the efficiency of absorption. Wheat bran has the potential to contribute to a condition known as 'leaky gut'. A leaky gut is one in which it becomes possible for substances that have not been fully digested to cross the intestinal wall and enter the bloodstream. This situation may be made worse by eating refined carbohydrates and processed sugar, which can encourage the growth of yeast organisms, which make the gut even more leaky. People with leaky guts are prone to allergies, skin conditions, low energy and weight gain.

Tea and coffee are digestion inhibitors. They reduce the availability of essential minerals including calcium, magnesium, zinc and iron. Tea and coffee are non-foods and are in fact classified as drugs. They have no nutritional status. Using these drugs over a prolonged period can have a significantly adverse influence on mineral status. Similarly, alcohol interferes with the absorption of magnesium, zinc and most B vitamins. Drinking tea, coffee and alcohol anywhere near a meal can undermine your ability to obtain essential nutrients that are needed for energy, immunity, hormone production and the health of your cells. Unfortunately, health warnings about tea, coffee and alcohol are not required and there is no warning on the label to tell you to avoid their consumption at least an hour either side of a meal.

In spite of what has been said about wheat bran (which should also contain a digestive health warning), inadequate fibre intake can diminish absorption in the small intestine by allowing a sticky goo to gum up the spaces between the villi. Low-fibre foods, especially those made from highly refined grains and carbohydrates, are particularly good at creating this sticky goo. So are animal products, including meat, dairy foods, fish and eggs. Not eating enough fibre reduces the intestine's ability to move food along and the sticky mess that results from a low-fibre diet can dramatically interfere with the absorption of many nutrients. This can lead to impacting of the intestines and consequently to serious bowel diseases. It slows down the whole movement along the intestine and hinders the digestive process. Eating plenty of fresh fruit and vegetables, whole grains and legumes, will help keep things moving along nicely. Soluble fibre, like that in oat bran or psyllium husks, is much better than the aggressive, unforgiving fibre in wheat bran.

The presence of toxic metals like lead, copper and mercury can directly block absorption of important minerals, including calcium and zinc. These can get into your food and water from contact with water pipes or cooking utensils. It is also an unfortunate fact that many fish are now contaminated with heavy metals, due to the industrial pollution of our seas and waterways. It only takes tiny amounts of these heavy metals to have negative effects on digestion. The absorption of minerals can also be hindered by taking tea, coffee and other stimulants or medications.

TUBE STOP 4 – COLON

Finally, in our journey on the tube, our digested food reaches the colon, a loop of intestine that ends up forming the stools that you pass as waste.

The colon is your very own waste disposal system. It turns the residues of food leaving the intestine into faeces ('poo' to you and me). The waste products remain in a semi-solid state and are moved slowly along the colon, being stored until they are removed from the body by going to the lavatory.

This part of the intestine is inhabited by millions of bacteria that perform some important tasks. These include helping you with immunity and with detoxification. They also make some vitamins (K, B12, thiamin and riboflavin). There are two main kinds of bacteria.

Bifidobacteria are 'friendly' bacteria which have a generally beneficial effect on health and bowel ecology. They produce mild acid and in some cases, B vitamins. These bacteria should be dominant in the gut.

Bacteriodes are potentially dangerous bacteria and if their presence increases to abnormally high levels they can cause problems. Up to about 15 per cent of overall flora presence is the safe limit for these putrefactive bacteria, which can give off toxic substances if they get too numerous. Putrefactive bacteria are encouraged by ingesting animal products, refined foods, stimulants and medications.

To help keep a positive balance of gut bacteria it is important to eat the right things in the right way and at the right time. Well-chewed, fresh, raw food preceding a meal will prepare the digestive system and quicken transit time through the tube. It introduces good fibre and key nutrients.

On the other hand, eating refined or very slow digesting foods (like a meat meal, sugar, dessert or white flour) can slow the passage of food and encourage predominance of the putrefactive, damaging bacteria.

For infants, breast-feeding is by far the best way to keep the gut flora healthy but, in our polluted environment, even this isn't always enough. Parents who have babies that don't sleep well are advised to consider giving them positive bacteria to help balance their baby's tiny gut and make the child more comfortable.

The use of antibiotics and steroids can interfere with bacterial activity and disrupt the balance of bad in favour of good. The frequent use of antibiotics, even a single course, can dramatically upset intestinal flora with significant problems for health.

Probiotics

Watch out for the big brand daily tubs of probiotics – they usually come in a dairy solution that is not ideal, and are often high in sugar which is counter-productive.

As a kick-start, a probiotic supplement and FOS (a substance that feeds good bacteria) is a useful addition to your intake.

Most people's tube systems are in negative bowel flora balance. This contributes to bad skin, lowered immunity, bloating, gas, nausea, fatigue, bad breath, headaches and joint pain. Excessive negative bacteria can produce toxins which are absorbed by the body, resulting in all of the above symptoms. They also potentially stimulate disease conditions due to the accumulation of morbid matter which cannot be readily eliminated.

Yeast infestations of the gut (encouraged by refined foods, alcohol and sugar) can penetrate the lining of the intestine. This penetration can make the intestinal wall more permeable than normal and allows undigested molecules, particularly partially digested proteins, through into the blood (the leaky gut I mentioned earlier). These molecules can then be recognized by the immune system, provoking an immune response. It is this immune response that then gives rise to the symptoms of allergy.

Keeping well hydrated (plenty of water), eating naturally fibrous foods (vegetables, whole grains and legumes), chewing well and eating slowly will all contribute to optimizing the health of the intestinal tube. This can speed up the normalization of weight, reduce allergies, improve skin, enhance rest from sleep, increase energy, improve immunity and give you positive feelings of well-being. Not to mention promoting an absence of bloating, leading to a flatter tummy and less gas!

FINAL TUBE STOP – EVERYBODY OUT!

Ideally you want your tube journey not to exceed twelve hours. You can test this out if you like. Eat a tin of sweetcorn (but don't chew too well just this time!) along with a meal. You should notice some corn kernels the next time you go to the lavatory. If you don't see them it is probable that your tube journey is taking too long.

Your bowels, when they are healthy, will move at least once a day. This is not the case for a scarily high number of people. Once or twice a day is ideal for the evacuation of your bowel. Stools should be soft, buoyant and break up on flushing. Many people are squeamish about urine and faeces: don't be. As you progress into eating real foods in the right way, you will find that your eliminations become progressively less offensive.

You are not what you eat. You are what you digest and absorb.

If you don't digest and absorb properly or thoroughly then you change your destiny. With every forkful, not just what you eat but how you eat it makes a difference to how you change and where you go.

Let's summarize what we've learned in this section. I make no apologies for the length of this: effective digestion is absolutely fundamental to your well-being. The health of your gut is closely linked with your brain. In fact your gut forms part of your mind. Where do you think the term 'gut feeling' comes from? Poor digestion can lead to stress and depression. Stress and depression interfere with the process of digestion. This is a powerful negative spiral.

To set your digestive spiral to the positive and get your gut and mind into balance there's a table over the page that sums up what you should do.

Give yourself the gift of powerful and perfectly balanced digestion

Objective:
To optimize the way in which your body is able to assimilate energy and intelligence from your environment by taking in nourishing food.

Benefits:
Feeling light, a leaner body, great mood, a feeling of balance and control, stronger immunity, more energy, positive outlook, greater general awareness, freedom from misplaced hunger. Less gas, flat tummy, comfortable digestion, more effective sleep. Vitality and well-being.

Strategies:

1. Drink a glass of water before any snack or meal.

2. Always start a meal with something fresh and raw (or lightly cooked) – a piece of fruit, a salad, a portion of vegetables.

3. Only start a meal when you are at level 1 on the satisfaction scale. Your stomach is completely empty and you cannot feel the presence of any food from a previous meal. There is a sensation of hunger. Real hunger for real food.

4. If you are tempted to eat when you are not at level 1, explore why. Don't eat but do something else. Even if everyone around you is eating and they accuse you of being on a diet. Tell them you just don't feel like eating right now. Focus on the friendship and conversation – have a glass of water and enjoy the sensation of every sip. Wonder at why your friends are eating when they don't need to – often at the same time as they discuss their cellulite, mood swings and lack of energy.

5. Never drink coffee or tea or alcohol within an hour of eating food. It prevents your digestion from getting full access to important nutrients.

6. Eat slowly. Enjoy every mouthful. Notice the feeling of digestion and the transport of energy and intelligence to your cells. Select foods that are full of energy and intelligence (more later about the difference between these and 'foods' that are lifeless and dumb).

7. Stop eating at level 4 – the point of optimum comfort – when you feel satisfied and there is neither hunger nor discomfort.

8. Do not attach feelings to foods. No matter how much the advertisers try to get you to. Take food at face value. Look at it critically. Smell it. Squeeze it between your fingers. Select foods that will help your body. Notice how they make your digestion feel.

9. Pay attention to your gut. Listen to what it tells you. Feel when it is comfortable. Notice when it doesn't feel great.

10. As far as you can, avoid eating refined foods: white flour, bread, cakes, biscuits, pasta, sugar, confectionery and chocolate.

BLOOD SUGAR – IF IT ISN'T IN BALANCE YOU HAVE A FRACTION OF THE ENERGY YOU SHOULD HAVE

Your body has a constant requirement for the right level of glucose in the bloodstream. You need to keep the equivalent of about a half-teaspoon of glucose in your blood at any one time. Your body is very sensitive to the amount of sugar in your blood and has sophisticated ways to keep the amount even. Too much glucose in your blood is dangerous – it can damage your nerves, eyes and kidneys.

Your brain needs a nice steady supply of glucose to operate effectively. Your body stores glucose in your liver so you always have a store nearby.

When you eat food, carbohydrates provide the glucose your body needs. Different foods release sugars at different rates. Some provide sugars that enter the bloodstream very fast. Others take more time. This is a very important distinction.

Because of this need for a constant supply of glucose, your body has evolved to like sweet foods. In the natural world, sweet foods are usually full of high energy and intelligence. The sweet foods are fruits, berries and root vegetables. They provide fresh, raw, living nourishment and plenty of vitamins. Other natural sources of carbohydrate are beans, pulses, whole grains and vegetables. All of these natural sources of carbohydrate bring with them the vitamins and minerals that are required to convert the energy they carry into a form that is usable by your body.

Refinement – a modern 'curse'?

But things have changed. A few hundred years ago some bright spark thought of the process of 'refinement'. The term 'refinement' was used to indicate the new products' purity; what were thought of as 'impurities' were removed. The major items to which 'refinement' was applied were wheat, rice and sugar.

Refinement was great. Refined grains were much less prone to attack by weevils and insects. Refined wheat lost the wheat germ that included its oils, and so did not go rancid in the holds of ships or in storehouses. The same goes for refined rice.

But refined sugar was in a class of its own. The pure white crystals were much prized. They appealed to the palate and became increasingly sought after. So much so that this new drug was peddled around the world in huge networks of trade that relied predominantly on slavery for production. Sugar was the first major drug trafficked globally. Whole empires were founded on it.

Refined grains and sugar are 'fast releasers'. When you eat them the sugar races into your blood. Your blood sugar rockets and your body's alarm bells ring. Your pancreas is instructed to produce insulin – a vital hormone – that adjusts your metabolism to extract the sugar from your blood and dump it, usually as fat on your buttocks, hips, belly, thighs and organs. The drop in blood sugar is rapid, so much so that it can, quite quickly, encourage your body to prompt you to eat again.

This blood sugar cycle is one of the most significant causes of the racing rates of obesity in our world. The use of refined grains, refined carbohydrates and sugar is literally killing us. It makes us fat, wears out our pancreas (which can lead to diabetes) and causes mental and emotional problems. Sugar and refined grains are potentially deadly.

So why aren't we taught this in school? Well, go back and read section one. Sugar and refined grains are one of the biggest monkey poles in modern nutrition. They are sold as food but they are not food. They have virtually no real nutritional value. They are empty of nourishment, providing only the illusion of nutrition because they deliver calories – 'pure', 'refined', 'empty' calories – but no vitamins, no minerals, no enzymes, no life, no nourishment. They strip your body of nutrients in order to be processed.

Not all calories are equal. Not all carbohydrates are equal

Refined sugar is a killer and the sugar pushers have created an entire framework of nutrition that has hoodwinked governments and consumers for over three hundred years. If you remember one thing from Livetetics remember this: sugar is a drug, a dangerous, potentially addictive drug. It is probably responsible for more deaths than any other substance on the planet and there is a lot of it about. In terms of health and the substance's knock-on effects, any government that is serious about drug trafficking should first place its hand on the shoulder of the sugar pushers. This, however, will take a long time to happen. The British empire was built on drug trafficking, starting with sugar and tea. These became institutionally acceptable because they were one of the foundations of the economy. They were never challenged and so the monkey pole was created.

Sugar and tea and coffee, like smoking, provide illusory benefits: the illusion of energy, the illusion of refreshment.

Look around you. Notice the little disclaimers that are popping up on labels. 'Please note that, like all soft drinks, product x should be drunk in moderation'. If you call them to ask what 'moderation' means you will be given a woolly answer. Notice the changes in slogans. The chocolate bar that once promised it would help you 'work rest and play' if you ate one every day now promises to deliver 'pleasure you can't measure'. A change in slogan to reach a new and changing market? Or a shift encouraged by the company's lawyers in the hope that lawsuits from obese and diabetic customers, who were dumb enough to actually eat one of those bars every day, might be avoided? My guess is that 'a chocolate bar a day helps you work rest and play' is a scientifically unsupportable proposition. Even with all the manipulation and distortion of science that takes place to further corporate interests, eventually the truth will out. Refined sugar's time is about to come. Our grandchildren will look back with horror at the appalling atrocity committed on humanity by the deceptive sale of refined sugar and other processed carbohydrates as 'food'.

Side effects

Constantly elevated blood sugar levels can have a number of rather nasty effects. It can mess up your heart and circulation. Cardiovascular complications include blockage or breakage of blood vessels in the heart, resulting in heart disease and strokes (arterial problems) and damage to kidneys, nerves or retinas (blood capillary problems). Elevated blood sugar is a constant risk factor in diabetes so these conditions are prevalent in diabetics. People who consistently eat refined carbohydrates and processed sugars are running the significant risk of wearing out their blood sugar management system, leading to full-blown diabetes. Then what might you have to look forward to?

Cataracts can result from the formation of sorbitol on the lens of the eye. Insoluble sorbitol crystals result from excess blood glucose and they become trapped in the lens. As the sorbitol concentration increases over time the osmotic pressure increases and the fluid drawn into the lens cells generates pressure that leads to cataracts.

The same sort of osmotic swelling can take place in peripheral capillaries resulting in poor circulation. This can open the way for gangrene (particularly in lower limbs) or the breakdown of filtration mechanisms in the kidney.

Elevated insulin from insulin injections is an attendant risk of diabetes. This predisposes to obesity by encouraging the conversion of glucose to fat.

Clearly the diabetic tending to obesity will increase the risks of cardiovascular disease. But you don't have to be diabetic to get this tendency to lay down fat. If you keep eating sugar and refined carbohydrates your system has to keep producing insulin and its frequent presence sets up the fat deposition pathways for you anyway. Sugar is a direct route to energy swings, mood swings and an excessively fat body.

Notice that the term 'a healthy balanced diet' is on the wane. Why? Because it is impossible to balance a diet that includes refined carbohydrates. These refined, 'empty' carbohydrates provide calories but no nourishment. Therefore they always have an anti-nutrition effect as we can't process them without using vitamins and minerals from elsewhere.

With modern foods containing fewer vitamins and minerals than ever before (up to 75 per cent less in some cases, according to official statistics), this means our nutrients are in short supply as it is. To try and use calories which don't bring any nourishment is like going to the pub with friends who don't bring any money. They just leach off you: and it makes you ill. And so the term 'balanced diet' is disappearing from the nutrition books and the 'varied diet' is in the ascendancy. It seems to be part of a semantic game that is played to deceive the legislators and consumers.

Stimulants vs supplements

Sugar and refined carbohydrates aren't the only culprits here. Stimulants like tea and coffee have negative effects on blood sugar. We know they are stimulants; they are drugs, just like sugar. They are foreign substances that have pharmacological effects. As this book is being written, there is legislation passing through the European Courts seeking to restrict the sale of nutritional supplements to 'safe' levels. There is, effectively, no evidence that there are any adverse effects reported from supplement products sold legitimately anywhere in Europe. But the legislation, designed to restrict the sale of safe and effective food supplements, will prevent consumers from having access to products that are beneficial to their health.

The legislation, however, is discriminatory because other food supplements, for which there is evidence of negative effects, are not included. So we find sales of certain vitamins are to be restricted but the sale of refined sugar (a chemical food supplement) is not to be affected. Sales of some mineral compounds will be outlawed but the sale of coffee, an addictive, damaging drug will continue to be allowed without health warnings. The law, as they say, is an ass. When it comes to definitions of food and the identification of what kills people, ignorruption is rife. The nutrition establishment is riddled with monkey poles. People are running around chanting the mantra, 'There is no such thing as an unhealthy food – only an unhealthy diet'. 'Everything in moderation' or 'a healthy varied diet' is all you need to be in good health, they claim. And most people believe them.

Some people are concerned when a 'food' is labelled 'bad' rather than 'good'. They find the distinction unhelpful. They think it has the potential to make people have trouble with food and experience disordered eating; to experience guilt and deprivation and then to fall off the rails and binge. My experience is exactly the opposite. I have found that in the majority of cases disordered eating arises when people do not know enough about food, the differences between foods and the effects that different foods have. Until we understand the difference between nourishment and anti-nutrition, of course we will experience disordered eating. Most people have disordered eating: they crave junk and they eat it. They get fat, they get sick, they die. That's pretty disordered!

Imagine yourself and three friends in 20–40 years time. Between the four of you, three will be dying of an unnecessary degenerative disease. The choice is yours. Well-being is available but your destiny is in your hands.

Cravings

If we eat foods that nourish us then our cravings subside. If we crave junk it is because we have misunderstood our hunger and, unless we know better, we expect the consumption of more junk to ease the hunger. But it fails. It is only by getting back in touch with our natural hunger, our healthy hunger, and by identifying positive, nourishing foods that satisfy our hunger (without the negative effects of blood sugar swings, excess fat, bloating, toxicity, mood swings or general ill-being) that we are then free of our slavery to junk. It is slavery to junk, and ignorance of the difference between foods and junk, along with chronic malnourishment, that leads to disordered eating.

So let's just accept it: sugar is not a food. Refined carbohydrates (white flour, biscuits, cake, and confectionery) are not food. A huge portion of what we consider a 'food group' is not food at all. It is just junk.

So, is there, in fact, a 'safe' or healthy level of refined sugar and other refined carbohydrates, as 'experts' would have us believe?

The short answer is no. According to Livetetic principles they are always negative and always damaging. They are to be treated with the utmost caution. The World Health Organization recommends that no more than ten per cent of your calories come from these empty sources. The sugar industry wants it to be 25 per cent.

Livetetics accepts that it is very hard to avoid refined carbohydrates altogether. If you have to use them then keep them to five per cent of your intake. And be sure to take a decent supplement and extra fresh, raw foods to make up for the anti-nutrition effects of the killer refined sugars.

Keeping your blood sugar even is one of the most important factors to ensure you keep fat off, energy high and minimize the risk of obesity, diabetes and heart disease. There are a number of things you can do:

Give yourself the gift of even blood sugar and consistent energy levels

Objective:
To supply your body with the energy sources it needs along with the nourishment and intelligence that will make a net gain rather than strip out existing reserves.

Benefits:
Reduction in cravings for junk. Consistent levels of energy through the day. A lean body. Improved digestion.

Strategies:

1. Eat regularly. Regular small meals and snacks are the order of the day. Eat something every hour or so with a 'meal' four or five times a day. But remember to only eat if you are at level 1. If you are comfortable then you can wait for your next meal.

2. Eating protein with your meals and snacks will assist your body in dealing with sugar. Things you should eat with each meal or snack are: tofu, beans, pulses, nuts, seeds, or a small quantity of chicken or fish.

3. Salads and vegetables. Eat a bowl of mixed salad twice a day. Use any salad you like and dress it with pure, unrefined vegetable oil. Also eat vegetables: broccoli, cauliflower and beans all make great additions either raw or lightly steamed.

4. Oat bran and fibre. This is delicious made into porridge with water or soya milk. Have it with some nuts and seeds. An excellent source of fibre, along with the fibre you'll be getting from your vegetables and salads which should all help your body deal with sugar more effectively.

5. Whole grains and whole carbohydrates. Always use whole grains and whole rice. These provide useful carbohydrates which come with vitamins and minerals that are needed to help process them.

6. Drink at least 8 glasses of pure, mineral water a day. It is very important to stay well hydrated. Drink two glasses on rising and a glass before each meal.

7. Significantly reduce or eliminate sugar and refined food. This may not be easy at first, but it needn't be difficult either. Just get rid of sugared foods and drinks. Replace them with regular snacks and meals that contain a good source of protein.

8. Avoid white bread, crackers, biscuits and cakes. These all have a rapid blood sugar effect.

9. Significantly reduce or eliminate tea, coffee and alcohol. These stimulants can ruin blood sugar balance and set up a negative blood sugar cycle.

10. Ensure there is a source of the mineral chromium in your diet and that your food intake delivers a good range of B vitamins and minerals.

DETOXIFICATION – CLEANING AWAY THE GARBAGE AND GETTING RID OF IT

O ur liver is our own fat-burning disposal unit. You will remember the journey along the tube. After your stomach, your beautifully chewed food made its way into the small intestine where it was spread very thinly over the thousands of villi. Elements of this digested food now travel across the walls of your villi and enter the bloodstream. First stop, the liver.

After picking up elements from the digestive process, all your enriched blood (if it is full of nutrients) or contaminated blood (if you have just eaten an empty carbohydrate food containing colourings, additives, pesticides and excess fat and salt) is pumped through the liver. The liver is a massive filter. It screens the blood from your intestine for all its contents, has fantastic potential to regenerate itself and expands as required (up to a point). It tries to regulate your blood: how much sugar is in it, how much fat is allowed through, proteins, hormones, everything. Your liver acts as the customs unit of your body by stopping 'travellers' who want to get in, checking potential immigrants for suitability and checking that returning travellers haven't contracted any diseases or brought home illicit or dangerous substances.

Security screen

Most toxic substances are immediately acted upon by the cells in your liver to de-activate them. Cells in your liver operate like millions of your own personal security guards and bomb disposal experts. They work tirelessly, 24 hours a day, trying to prevent terrorists from getting into your open bloodstream with dangerous objects that can damage and kill your cells.

Your liver has to deal with any toxins created by the process of digestion. As we have already learned these toxic by-products are dramatically increased if we eat sugar with our food because it encourages acid fermentation in the gut and promotes the growth of negative bacteria and yeasts.

There are the normal toxic by-products of digestion to deal with and there are toxins from non-foods, better known as junk. And so your liver has to deal with toxic rubbish from coffee, alcohol, nicotine, medical drugs, food additives, pesticides, colourings and flavourings. It is worth noting that there is virtually no difference between 'artificial' or 'natural' flavours and colours. Use of the term 'natural' simply demands that the raw material includes some plant source: the final chemical additive is virtually the same. So statements like 'free from artificial additives' are really marketing ploys: you must still read the label to see if additives are used. The colouring and flavouring of food is simply a way for manufacturers to fool you into believing something that looks and tastes strange is actually good enough to eat. If possible, you should avoid any coloured or flavoured food; they have been designed to trick your natural senses.

If your liver could operate with 100 per cent efficiency and completely screen and clean your blood, it is possible that you would never age or at least, age far, far more slowly than you might. And that is your liver's objective. To keep your blood and body tissues optimally clean, full of nutrients and clear of waste.

You already know how sugar and refined carbohydrates can set up the blood sugar see-saw; rapid rises followed by rapid drops and the resultant establishment of cravings for yet more junk. The liver helps to regulate this process along with your pancreas and your adrenals. The adrenals secrete hormones that stimulate the liver to release glycogen (stored carbohydrates) and so put glucose in the blood if glucose gets too low.

Your pancreas secretes insulin when blood sugar is too high and this encourages the liver to store glucose. This is fine as long as the glucose warehouse in the liver is not full. Once the liver's stores are full then the sugar has to be converted into fat. And fat has to be dumped. It starts around your liver and then your other organs and eventually fat just starts sticking to you everywhere. Especially to the parts that don't move very much: your belly, your buttocks, your hips, your breasts.

Your system is designed so that the regulation of blood sugar should be smooth and even with enough glycogen stored to keep you going if you don't eat. You should be able to go for several days without eating and not experience any major symptoms of high or low blood sugar levels.

But, our brains operate better at slightly elevated blood sugar levels and we get the impression of feeling better when glucose is slightly up. In the quest for this sugar 'high', our food-junkie society has found a host of ways to push up blood sugar, and so we eat refined sugar, white flour products and chocolate, drink coffee, carbonated sugar water and alcohol, take drugs and go for excitement (sugar via the adrenals). Emotional stress, bizarrely, can also raise our blood sugar, so some of us even get into a cycle of making ourselves feel bad so we can get the illusion of feeling good, in a negative sort of way. Others engage in 'extreme' sports or adventures to get their sugar 'high'.

Other functions of the liver

Regulation of fats is another critical function of your liver. If you want to adjust your fat deposits, even get rid of them, then your liver is the organ to love and look after. A stressed and toxic liver cannot manage fat properly; it cannot effectively deal with massive sugar swings and it cannot effectively screen the blood for 'terrorists'. You need to treasure your liver if you want effective fat loss and sensible regulation of your body.

Another important job of your liver is to regulate hormones. Hormones are little chemical messengers that one part of the body sends to another to get a result. They travel through the bloodstream in a heartbeat and visit cells to tell them what to do. You already know about insulin, the hormone that is sent to get sugar out of your blood and store it as glycogen or fat (these days, usually fat). Hormones are essential to keep your body in balance. But if hormones were allowed to keep flowing around your system their messages would become out of date and there would be utter confusion. Your liver processes hormones and breaks them down so that redundant messages no longer get around the system.

If your liver is overloaded and sluggish this hormone processing can become impaired and hormones are allowed to keep running around the system, upsetting the body's balance. An example of this is seen in men who have livers damaged by half a lifetime of macho beer drinking sessions, consumption of refined carbohydrates and excess fat from animal products. They run the serious risk of developing fatty deposits on their chests, as breasts. It is ironic that consumption habits commonly thought of as macho – eating meat, drinking alcohol and caring little for food quality – can have such a feminine outcome!

Toxic stresses on the liver

This hormone-processing capability is even more important today than it was 50 years ago. Our food and environment is riddled with chemicals that mimic hormones. Pesticide residues, food additives, industrial pollutants and growth hormones used to fatten up animals, are all in the food chain. These substances only need to exist in almost unimaginably small quantities to make a big difference in our bodies. Some of them sneak through our liver's defences and exert hormonal effects on our bodies. Others would normally be made safe – held up on entry – but our livers are so exhausted by trying to deal with the metabolic poisons from our bad food choices that they simply can't cope with the extra demands.

Signs of hormonal imbalance in women – the bloating, breast tenderness and mood changes of premenstrual syndrome – are symptoms that usually vanish altogether with improvements in liver function.

Animal foods provide the most toxic stress on the liver. Meat from cattle force-fed with unnatural feeds and injected with antibiotics and growth hormones can be riddled with toxic debris. Not to mention the negative emotional energy of a stressful life and a violent death. Deep-water fish, all over the planet, are contaminated with heavy metals, pesticides and other industrial pollutants. Many of the manufacturers who now ask us to trust them with their technological mutation of plants and animals through genetic modification have been responsible for the permanent pollution of this beautiful planet with their noxious compounds.

Excessive protein consumption from meat and dairy products, combined with refined carbohydrates that cause acid fermentation in the gut, putrefactive bacteria and yeasts, is a common source of the liver overload we experience: this is before we have even thought about dealing with the drug residues from coffee, tea, alcohol and chocolate, which then swill around with pesticides, food colourings, chemical flavourings and preservatives.

Our liver bears the brunt. It is an incredible machine performing over 500 vital functions. But it has limits. Your liver is a potential powerhouse. Because of its hormone processing function it acts as a kind of metabolic MC. It is the main regulator of the blood and is a fundamental key to finding and charging your metabolic rate. To charge up your metabolism you need to improve the liver. You improve the liver by improving digestion and you improve liver function by removing unnecessary toxic stress in the food you eat.

> *You do not become healthier by losing weight. You lose weight by becoming healthier.*

In the same way that your body knows what temperature it should be, your body knows exactly what weight you should be. Get your liver in shape and your body will regulate itself beautifully. Do not waste time worrying about what weight you should be according to some ridiculous 'standard' or 'fashion'. Rather use how you feel as a measure of your success. As your increased vitality begins to shine through, you will find that by aiming for health and well-being your true beauty and weight control will become automatic. Your liver is your own, personal fat disposal unit, if it has enough potential for running at its optimum capacity.

Excess weight is a symptom of imbalanced and impaired body function. Among the most important of these is the function of your liver. Your liver affects how you feel and how you feel affects how you behave: another spiral, a spiral of decline if it's negative and a spiral of ascendancy if it's positive. It is critical to set up a positive spiral. How pointless to treat depression with antidepressant drugs that even further stress the liver. How futile to treat 'women's troubles' with extra hormones that further stress the liver. How ridiculous to treat a toxic headache with pain killers that provide yet more toxic burden.

In spite of all of its brilliance – we have to acknowledge it – modern medicine so often completely misses the point. It is futile to treat symptoms unless the underlying cause is known and addressed. To treat a headache without treating the cause of the headache is just a short-term fix. To treat indigestion without sorting out the cause of the indigestion is pointless. To cut out a piece of bowel without addressing the cause of the rupture is again just taping over the problem. Modern medicine is too concerned with the symptom, and not the cause.

Look at the box opposite – it makes a very telling point.

What you would do is probably very different to what is happening, in terms of policy, in modern medicine and the way it is set up and run. Why does so much of modern medicine ignore the basic and well-known causes of degenerative disease? If heart disease is related to diet and lifestyle, if diabetes and obesity are created by the way we eat and live, if cancer is significantly (if not totally) driven by our diet and lifestyle, then why is this not addressed much more fully than it is?

I suggest there are two reasons:

1) There is money to be made by selling you junk as food. Junk is easy to make. It lasts a long time without going off. It is easy to transport. People like it and will buy it. You can easily add chemicals and drugs to junk to trick people into making them believe it tastes good. The profit margins are high. You can sell what consumers want: taste, convenience, and indulgence.

2) There is money to be made by treating the symptoms created by the consumption of junk sold as food. Degenerative diseases like diabetes, heart disease, cancer, osteoporosis, all send the cash tills ringing. Once you get a victim of degenerative disease in your clutches, you can sell them drugs for life.

And so the food manufacturers create their vehicles for deception. Foundations, Associations, Councils, Institutes, Research Centres and Charities, are all designed to position their 'foods' as safe and wholesome. All fine, as long as they are eaten as part of a 'healthy varied diet'.

Chant with me the food industry mantra: 'There is no such thing as an unhealthy food, only an unhealthy diet'.

This is the crux of Livetetics. Livetetics says there *are* unhealthy 'foods', and very unhealthy ones at that (see page 138, 'Foods versus drugs').

The pharmaceutical and medical equipment manufacturers keep promoting the idea that they are helping us by treating and curing our diseases. The doctor is established by common belief as the only person who knows what goes on inside your body. Yet just look at the way medical specialization has gone: endocrinologists specialize in hormones;

gastroenterologists specialize in digestion; psychologists specialize in the mind; cardiologists specialize in the heart; immunologists specialize in immunity; dermatologists specialize in skin. Round and round we go, not once looking at the body as a whole and whether or not it is 'in tune' and balanced.

In my clinical practice I have encountered specialists who deal with hormone disorders, who are not aware in any real way of the impact of their patients' livers on their condition. I have met psychiatrists who ignore the relationship of the digestive system to mind and mood. I have met surgeons who remove lumps and abscesses and who do not then give their patients any advice, or mis-advice, on how to prevent their recurrence.

Bad people? Ignorant people? By no means, just victims of the way it is. Unable to see the wood for the trees, bound by the limits of the framework of their education, many of them excellent practitioners, doing their best with all good intention. Sometimes, when the obvious relationships between different body systems are brought to their attention, they are interested to learn more. Sometimes they are totally dismissive. Some doctors, when they learn of the extent of the role of nutrition in health, are fascinated and they go on to study it more. Others are just too stuck in the deep rut of their education to see over the edge.

Meet the 'food people'

I have experienced the same with the food people. I used to be cynical and angry and think they were all con men. But over the last couple of years my nutrition consultancy has been treating the most senior managers in one of the world's largest food manufacturers. They are lovely people. They are bright and enthusiastic and really have the well-being of their company at heart. There are, as you would expect, also a few belligerent, rude, old men as well (toxic livers, perhaps) who would have nothing to do with our consultants or their advice. But, on the whole, the individuals in these organizations are consistently trying to do what consumers want, understand their needs and meet them. They know that this is what is good for business.

We treat these managers with diet and food supplements. They get to look and feel much better. For the most part they are completely ignorant, in their own lives, of the extent of the fundamental role that food and nutrition plays in their own health and well-being. Many are very surprised at the results. Following my nutrition consultants' advice has helped managers in this huge international food company to lose weight, gain more energy, lower cholesterol, improve digestion, gain better skin condition and be more productive. The results are clear.

But what is the response of members of their scientific and nutrition community? Outrage! Outrage that senior managers would consult with a nutrition organization that believes additional nutrients (above the Recommended Daily Amounts) can be beneficial to health; that they could entertain as credible a nutrition organization that would suggest reductions in dairy and sugar consumption as a path to well-being.

Most of the senior managers in this company are genuinely ignorant of the effects of their products. Most of their nutrition community is hamstrung by the limits of their education and experience.

Ignorruption

There are drug companies that knowingly sell dangerous chemicals that make things worse instead of better. There are beauty companies that sell worthless lotions and potions that do not work and, in many cases, make things worse. And there are food manufacturers that sell damaging junk as food without giving consumers the information they need to make an informed decision.

There are industry bodies that would have us believe their products are essential in a healthy diet. To the extent that their lobbying has convinced governments to recommend that everyone eat from their 'food group' every day, even though there is plenty of evidence that eating from that 'food group' is not only unnecessary but downright dangerous (and deadly for many).

So, if reading about your liver and accepting that it can be responsible for a huge portion of your ailments, including your being excessively fat, is news to you, then be gentle on yourself. Most people aren't aware of this information. It is perfectly possible to become a medical doctor without the slightest clue as to what is going on with nutrition. There are still medical communities that debate whether diet has any more than a superficial role in disease.

Of course, to a certain extent this debate is necessary. After all, what would happen to the pharmaceutical industry if people learned about the power of food and nutrition and started to suffer less from degenerative disease?

Nutritional supplementation

What might happen, for example, if it was discovered that nutritional supplementation was becoming widespread? That consumers were becoming better informed and wanted to take a more proactive role in their health and well-being; and that this increasing practice of gaining extra nutrition through supplementation had the potential to threaten downstream revenues from the sale of chemical treatments for degenerative diseases?

Well, here's what's happening in Europe.

Some bright spark raises an issue at the EU and suggests that nutritional supplements are harmful. There is no evidence that this is the case but a collection of 'experts' raises it. (Bear in mind that the pharmaceutical lobby is one of the most powerful lobbies in Europe.)

And so a group is set up to look at the issue. The group is mandated to look at all the evidence and come up with rules about what may and may not be sold to consumers as food supplements. A list of nutrients is created and the 'expert' group begins to look at the 'research', which is a rather limited band of research that looks only at possible evidence of toxicity. They don't find much, and what little they do find has already been challenged and discredited in previous national investigations of the same subject.

Yet stalwartly and resolutely, the legislation is pushed through. The list of 'acceptable' supplements is restricted; the levels that are 'acceptable' are reduced and so consumers are about to be prevented from making safe and effective choices that will improve their health and well-being.

Is the EU commissioner responsible for this process corrupt? Is he taking back-handers from pharmaceutical companies? Is he ignorant? Is he really completely unaware of the stupidity of the process and the limits of its credibility? Or is he just ignorrupt, a good guy setting out to do something worthwhile? No one is against clear labelling, safe products, and quality ingredients, which is the mandate of his expert group. But it has been conceived in such a way that it does not look at the big picture, does not weigh up the benefits and does not look at all the evidence.

Reclaim responsibility for yourself

And so it is up to us, the individuals, to take responsibility. To stand back and look at the landscape. To see the interaction of things and hear the silent messages that whisper to us when we listen for them. To read the hidden messages that tumble out from between the lines and notice what we didn't notice before.

We cannot rely on the law, the government, the committees, the organizations, the companies, the federations or any other collections of interests, for they are riddled with ignorance, good intention, stupidity, competence, incompetence, honesty and corruption, and it is very difficult to tell which is dominant in any group. Ignorruption is rife.

You have to look out for yourself.

The normal way for you to feel is positive, cheerful, stable and energetic. When the liver gets clogged up then people start to feel pessimistic, irritable, depressed and experience rapid mood fluctuations, one moment high and another down in the dumps.

'Grumpy old man', 'stroppy old bat', 'time of the month', 'miserable as sin'. But only one description usually is required: 'toxic liver'.

Is it really possible that our technologically advanced western medicine could overlook such a common problem as a toxic liver? Yes, easily! Diagnosis in western medicine is based mainly on tissue condition. If what is being examined shows no sign of damage then it is considered not to be a problem. Blood tests, scans, x-rays, have been developed to pick up damaged states. The real issue, though, is energy and balance. If we can establish, maintain and restore energy and balance then tissue damage is much less likely. Finding tissue damage and then labelling the damage as a 'condition' or a 'disease' is to ignore the actual cause of the condition.

And so, when we test the liver in modern medicine we examine the blood for enzymes that belong in the liver. No enzymes: liver assumed OK. Enzymes: indication of ruptures and problems in the liver. So liver 'function' tests don't actually examine function at all; they identify damage. Unfortunately for the patient with early-stage liver function problems, their ailments (bad skin, mood swings, fat arms, cellulite, low energy) are put down to something else and 'treated' as conditions of their own. So we take medications to ease our symptoms, further stress our livers and wait until we have a rupture. Then, at last, we can find the cause of our 'disease'.

So what are you going to do? Well one suggestion is not to fall into the river or to keep away from the edge of the cliff. Once you've slipped in it can be the devil of a job to scramble back. But it can be done! It is never too late. Your body is an extraordinary thing and your capacity for healing and regeneration is unprecedented. The most powerful healing forces are already in your body. You were created with them and they are always there. You know it.

Start achieving

I suggest that you set a goal. Perfect health and well-being. A perfect body – perfect for you – your unique, perfect body (not what some young advertising executive tells you your body should be). Set out on a quest for your own truth, your own reality, what works for you. Look around you for examples of success and follow them. Find practitioners who are well. Find teachers whom you respect. Read books written by people who care for you. Prepare your own food.

There have been times when you felt incredibly strong. Our lives are peppered with examples of people who survive under the most incredible circumstances, and who pull themselves back from the most ghastly of disease states.

Set your goal and find a way to achieve it.

You're on the path. Take a deep breath, and another one. Drink a glass of water. Do it now!

Did you drink the glass of water?

If 'yes' you made a decision that will change your destiny.

If 'no' you made a decision that won't change your destiny.

Your choice.

Your destiny.

Your responsibility.

Give yourself the gift of a clean, healthy, productive liver

Objective:
To ensure my liver is able to perform, with perfect efficiency and effectiveness, the critical functions necessary to clear my blood of waste, manage fat, protect me from poisons, feed and nourish my cells and tissues.

Benefits:
More energy, positive outlook, elation, freedom from pain, feeling lighter, being leaner, greater sexual potency, looking young for my age, enhanced immunity.

Strategies:

1. Always start the day with a glass of water, ideally, with a freshly squeezed lemon in it. This can be warm if you like. Sip it while you breathe deeply. This sets up your digestive system.

2. Focus on eating plenty of the cruciferous vegetables along with high vegetable and fruit intake. These aid detoxification. Broccoli and cauliflower must feature regularly in your meals.

3. Focus on whole foods that bring their own nutrients with them. These are digested more effectively and provide living health and energy to the digestive process.

4. Eat fresh, raw and lightly cooked foods that are prepared just before you eat them. Follow all the strategies that deliver effective digestion.

5. Lie down for 10 minutes three times during the day. Outside if you can. Getting horizontal flushes the liver with blood and helps the detoxification process.

6. Brushing your skin with a soft to medium bristle brush helps clear dead skin and allows it to operate as a channel of elimination for debris. Enhance this by taking an alternating hot and cold shower after brushing, to boost blood flow under the skin, get circulation moving and encourage elimination and regeneration.

7. Move and exercise gently every day for a consistent 30 minutes. Make sure the exercise raises your heart rate and increases depth of breathing but does not make you out of breath. This stimulates digestion and circulation, both of which make the liver's job easier.

8. Avoid eating sweet foods with any meal. This sets up acid fermentation and produces unnecessary toxic wastes.

9. Eliminate drugs, stimulants and pollutants that add toxic load to the liver, such as tea, coffee, alcohol, chocolate, caffeinated drinks and over-the-counter medications. Eat uncontaminated food, avoiding chemical food additives and pollutants including artificial sweeteners, colourings, flavours, preservatives and pesticide residues.

10. Avoid animal foods including meat, chicken and dairy products. Because these are at the top of the food chain, they are almost always riddled with pollutants and modern husbandry leaves them contaminated with hormones, antibiotics and pesticides.

ENERGY AND METABOLISM – YOUR INTERNAL FURNACE AND ENERGY PRODUCTION PLANTS

Have you ever tried to light a fire, a wood fire in a fireplace, a camp fire or a barbecue? It starts with a flame. One little flame will create a nice strong fire if you have small dry tinder to get it going. Once you have a strong flame then you are able to put on some bigger twigs and small logs. Little by little you can get the heat up, grow the flame until, eventually, you are able to put on coal or large logs and they will burn merrily.

Ever tried to light a slightly damp log with a match?

You don't stand a chance. It's just a waste of a box of matches and you're likely to burn your fingers.

Inside your body are around 75 trillion little fires burning. Each cell has its own energy production plant. These little powerhouses produce energy and heat by processing nutrients. A by-product of the process is the giving off of waste residues. If these little furnaces burn good clean fuel and you keep them well stoked up, and regularly clean away the burned residues and the waste products they give off, then they are a fabulous source of vitality and well-being.

But if you try to burn rubbish in them, then your little furnaces still do their best, but they are going to have reduced output and will give off smoke and other noxious waste. Ever tried throwing a rubber tyre on a bonfire? It burns all right, but it gives off foul, choking black smoke. Sure, it might give off some heat, but you're left with a bad taste in your mouth and a filthy black mess to clear away where the tyre once was.

It's not the quantity of calories – it's the QUALITY of calories that counts

Most of us do not pay much attention to how we feed our fires. Some of us have got as far as working out that food provides energy. We have been taught that we can measure the 'energy' in a food by working out how much energy it would give off if you burned it. We call the units of this energy 'calories'; different foods provide different amounts of calories.

If you've ever been on a diet, it will have almost certainly suggested that you reduce the overall number of calories in your intake. But what most of us were never told was that all calories are not equal. There is nice clean, efficient energy and there is foul, black, smelly, smoky 'energy'.

Quality calories

It is your responsibility to put clean fuel in your engine. And it begins with your stomach and digestion. Most people have a stomach that is a shadow of its potential. It spends most of its time in spasm and shock as it needs an inbound supply of clean, fresh, easily-digested food that has been eaten slowly and thoroughly chewed – which rarely happens. Feed the cells in your digestive system well and they will produce energy – the more energy the better you digest, the better you digest the more energy – a wonderful positive spiral.

But most of us have damp, flickering, digestive flames and instead of nurturing and kindling that flame we dump big lumps of garbage on to it and expect it to burn. It doesn't; it just does what it can to pass the garbage through as safely as possible. This costs energy – and your digestive system needs a lot of energy to function well – and so a negative spiral is set up.

So, the quality of the fuel you eat is one of the most important drivers of the quality of your metabolism. Your metabolism is your energy production plant. The coordinated attempt of your entire body to produce the energy you need for absolute vitality and well-being. 75 trillion little power plants fed via the furnace of your digestive system.

Now, most people think that energy is energy is energy. This is one of

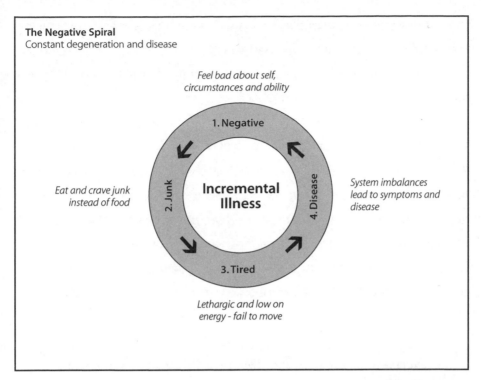

The Negative Spiral
Constant degeneration and disease

*Feel bad about self,
circumstances and ability*

1. Negative

2. Junk

**Incremental
Illness**

4. Disease

*Eat and crave junk
instead of food*

*System imbalances
lead to symptoms and
disease*

3. Tired

*Lethargic and low on
energy - fail to move*

the biggest lies in nutrition today. A few weeks ago a government minister was interviewed on the radio. She was being asked why the nation was becoming so rapidly obese and wouldn't it be a good idea for the government to intervene by trying to ensure we ate a healthier diet? Her response was that she didn't think the government getting involved in diet was a good idea; it would smack of a 'nanny' state. But, she said, and I quote: 'The reason we are overweight is that we do not do enough exercise – we are eating the same number of calories that we always have.' My children laughed and laughed. They might not be government ministers but they at least know the difference between foods and the difference between calories. And they know how different calories are today, compared with the way they used to be. It makes my children howl with laughter when they hear government ministers make stupid statements that are straight out of the PR manual given to them by the nutrition bodies set up by the food manufacturers. The quality of our calories gets lower and lower all the time and it is this primarily – as well as lack of exercise – that is creating the obesity epidemic (go to page 146 for a diagram that illustrates this point more fully).

What does this mean for 'calorie-controlled diets'?

We need calories for energy – right? That's what we've been taught. We need a certain number of calories each day to stay alive. Eat more than we need, we get fat. Eat less than we need, we get thinner. That's what we've been taught. We need to count calories. Eat less, lose weight. Eat more, gain weight. But look at the box below. It makes a very good point; one which shows that how the majority of people 'diet' to lose weight is flawed from the start.

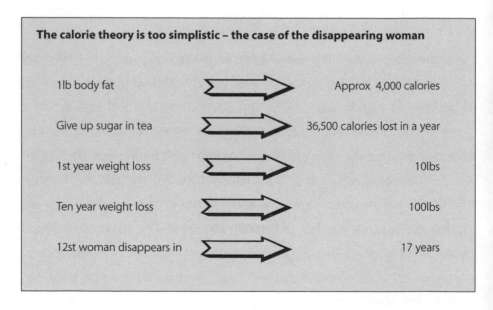

The calorie theory is too simplistic – the case of the disappearing woman

1lb body fat	→	Approx 4,000 calories
Give up sugar in tea	→	36,500 calories lost in a year
1st year weight loss	→	10lbs
Ten year weight loss	→	100lbs
12st woman disappears in	→	17 years

We'll talk more about this later, but these confused yet widely perpetuated ideas about calories demonstrate a total misunderstanding of what is going on inside the body.

Exercise is, of course, an issue. But one of the primary reasons nobody does any exercise is that they are so tired and lethargic that they can't get their backsides out of their chairs long enough to make a cup of tea let alone go and play a game, ride to work, walk the kids to school or get active in the garden.

In the same way that you can't lose weight until you are healthier, you cannot exercise effectively unless you have energy. The negative spiral is to eat junk, suppress the energy of your digestive system, pollute your cellular powerplants and so reduce your energy. So if you are a non-exerciser, stop feeling bad. Just as being fat isn't your fault, and being diseased isn't your fault, not exercising isn't your fault either.

Yes, I am suggesting that it is nobody's fault that they are fat, sick or inactive. It is however, your total responsibility.

How fat, well or active you are is 100 per cent your responsibility and your choice. So why isn't it your fault? How can that be?

It isn't your fault because you have been misled. Consistently and thoroughly misled throughout your entire life by people like the government minister who made that stupid comment on the radio. But many of these people probably thought they were telling the truth. So are they liars or are they just mistaken? I've given up trying to work out the difference, but what I do believe is that you cannot be responsible for your health unless you are given the information you need to make effective decisions. Once you have this information then you have freedom then you have choice and then you can exercise responsibility.

Are you an addict?

Want to jump out of aeroplanes and fall to the ground dangling beneath a parachute? Go ahead.

Want to ski jump off the top of a mountain? Go ahead.

Want to dive deep under the ocean and explore dark caves? Go ahead.

People do these things in spite of the fact that they are potentially dangerous. They do them often because they are dangerous. Remember we are sugar junkies by nature and our lives are tame compared with the world we evolved in. Stimulating adrenal stress is one way for people to get kicks, a hormonally induced glucose 'high'.

Want to take drugs to give yourself the short-term illusion that you feel better? Go ahead.

Most people who come to me wanting a better life are surprised when I tell them they are drug addicts. They look at me in a peculiar sort of way and then expect me to retract the statement. But I don't.

I have parents who bring five-year-old children into my office and these children are drug addicts. They are hopelessly addicted to powerful, addictive substances.

The parents don't like the thought that their children are drug addicts. They expect me to be using the term as a metaphor, as just a way of making a point.

However, the reality is that you are a probably a drug addict. If you are not a drug addict, and you are reading this book to reinforce what you already know, then forgive me. But most people are drug addicts so I'm on pretty safe ground.

We know that smoking tobacco is drug addiction. But most smokers don't think of themselves as drug addicts or 'junkies'. Is there a difference between the heroin addict and the tobacco addict? Not much, from a biochemical point of view. They both shoot poisonous substances direct into their bloodstreams, by-passing the protection of their digestive systems. One junkie does so by injection, the other by inhalation. They do it ostensibly to 'feel better'. The primary difference, of course, is that the tobacco junkie can use his drug legally and the heroin junkie cannot. One drug can be bought in reputable retail outlets and the other can't. One is socially acceptable and the other is not.

Alcohol is similar. This time the drug is taken by mouth but it is able to pass quickly into the bloodstream and it rapidly crosses the natural defences in the brain, where it can easily by-pass the blood brain barrier to interfere with brain processes and give the illusion of enhanced relaxation and well-being.

I don't believe prohibition works. People need crutches to get through life and they should be free to find their own way. I agree that behaviour that may be offensive or dangerous to others should be discouraged or prevented but, otherwise, freedom is the grand thing.

So I agree in a small way with our government minister about not becoming a 'nanny' state when it comes to food. People don't respond well to being told what to do by someone else: I know I don't. And legislative action tends to be ineffective anyway: there will always be a way around it. Ban tobacco advertising and sports sponsorship rockets; ban advertising to children and they'll find another way, through sponsoring school 'education' programmes or some other irresponsible and underhand technique.

The solution? Self-reference and information.

I suggested just now that you were probably a drug addict. If you smoke you might accept this. If you drink alcohol regularly you might not quite accept it. Tobacco and alcohol are fairly obvious drugs. However, whether you do or do not drink alcohol or smoke, the likelihood is that you are an addict of some substance or other.

'Aha – he's talking about tea and coffee', you may be thinking. Well, to a certain extent yes, I am. There are a great many habitual drinkers of tea and coffee. These commodities contain known drugs and they are taken to stimulate illusions of well-being in exactly the same way that crack cocaine, heroin and, indeed, tobacco and alcohol are taken. Is there any difference between tea and crack cocaine? They are not entirely dissimilar. Tea (or alcohol) is different in that it is a drug that has social acceptability. It is sold as food: coffee and tea are sold alongside foods, as foods. Yet they provide virtually no nourishment at all. They simply provide a few milligrams of known drugs that are taken deliberately for their 'uplifting' or 'relaxing' or 'mood enhancing' effect.

If you are a tea and coffee drinker you probably don't consider yourself a drug addict. If you drink it habitually then you almost certainly are.

Foods versus drugs

Let's get down to it: what is the difference between a 'food' and a 'drug'? It is an interesting and incredibly important question, and there are a lot of people fighting about this distinction. So let's cut through it all and give you a Livetetic definition:

A food provides nourishment for body function and well-being.

A drug is a substance that provides an illusion of well-being with effectively no nourishment and/or the possibility of depleting us of nourishment or stressing our body systems in some way.

When we talk about 'nourishment' in Livetetics we mean a collection of essential nutrients, fibre, living energy and natural intelligence.

Therefore, tobacco, alcohol, tea and coffee are clearly drugs. Interesting to note, though, that in spite of the known dangers of drinking coffee the product does not carry any useful labelling of caffeine content, any dosage information, any indication of maximum consumption and no warnings of the known side-effects. Consumers are expected to 'just know' these somehow. There is legislation about food supplements currently going through the European Courts, which demands clear labelling, clear information about contents and clear warnings about any potential overdose. However coffee, a clear non-food, is excluded from the process – why is this?

Because the process of government and legislation is riddled with ignorance, corruption and ignorruption. The coffee loophole is probably a combination of all three.

So, you don't smoke, you don't drink alcohol, you don't drink tea and coffee; now you're in the clear, aren't you? No, I'm afraid you're not.

Understanding the myth

Let's now deliver the answer to our health crisis. It is an answer that will come out over the next two generations. It will take that long because of the arguments that will occur between food manufacturers, legislators and scientists. But Livetetics gives the answer to you now.

You are being sold drugs as food. And you are addicted to them. You are a drug addict.

The most pernicious of these drugs is refined sugar. Sugar's chemical form is that of a carbohydrate and it contains 'calories'. But it contains no nourishment. Sugar has never been a food, never will be, and has no place being sold as food.

Sugar is a drug. It is an addictive drug and it kills people. It kills them with obesity, diabetes, heart disease and a myriad of other related 'diseases'.

Sugar provides an illusion. An illusion of taste, energy and well-being. One of the reasons it is so potent as a drug is that we have an evolutionary craving for sweetness. We've already talked about this. Now we're going to talk about it some more. Because we're talking about energy, about our 75 trillion power plants, and about giving those cells what they need to thrive and survive rather than to wilt and die.

Refined sugar contains calories but it does not contain energy.

Let me repeat that.

Refined sugar contains calories but it does not contain energy.

This is very important and it is a statement with which a lot of people disagree. For the most part they are the people that make and sell sugar. Other people who disagree are those who have been taught by the people that make and sell sugar. And then there are the ignorrupts – the people who believe both these groups.

Actually, it's very obvious. The notion that sugar contains energy is an illusion but it's not even a very good one. My six-year-old daughter understands it but the heads of most of the UK's nutrition bodies do not. Sugar contains calories and… NOTHING ELSE.

Let's take a look at how we convert calories to energy. Each of these little power plants of ours has to create energy; the cells in our bodies need to stay alive. They have functions to perform: to make skin or grow hair, or make hormones or fight germs, or any of a million other tasks depending on where and what it is. Cells need energy and, for the most part, have to make their own.

To make energy, these cells need carbohydrate. They take it and, through a series of chemical reactions, they convert it into energy in the presence of oxygen.

For this series of reactions to take place, vitamins, minerals and enzymes are required. Some the body has to get from the outside via the food we eat, and some can be made. The ones that can be made need other vitamins, minerals and enzymes for their reaction streams.

Now let's imagine you eat a food that consists of refined sugar or part-refined sugar. This presents the body with an illusion of energy, an illusion of food. Sugar is a carbohydrate and it can race through the digestive system and get into the blood. We've already discussed how this causes a hormonal response that sets up a cycle of cravings and adjusts your metabolism to dump carbohydrates as fat. But this is only one aspect of this drug's vicious effects.

To consume a carbohydrate in the absence of the nourishment needed to process it has an overall negative effect on your nutritional status. To process sugar you need vitamins, enzymes, minerals and a host of nourishment that we haven't even discovered yet. Refined sugar brings no nourishment with it. In this way it could be called an anti nutrient because, to process it, the body has to get nutrients and resources from elsewhere.

We've talked about this before and you'll remember how we described refined foods (those that provide calories with little or no nourishment) as leeches. Like drinking with the friend who invites you to the pub but takes no money of his own, you end up having to pay; with sugar and refined foods you pay with your life.

You need to understand, and understand well, that 'energy' when it is written on the side of a 'food' packet does not necessarily mean what it says. It may indicate the number of 'calories' that a chemist measures in the contents of the packet but it does not indicate anything about the nourishment of the food.

So parents happily give bottles and cartons of sugar water to their children thinking they are giving them 'energy',

> *You are being sold drugs as food: there is, therefore, such a thing as an 'unhealthy' food*

when they are actually sucking the life right out of them. Shelves in supermarkets are not just full of colas and sugar sodas, they are now full of 'sports' refreshment concoctions and 'energy' drinks to which paltry amounts of vitamins and amino acids have been added. But as long as they contain refined and processed sugar they are anti-nutrients and anti-energy.

Yet, when my son crosses the box in his SAT science paper confirming the statement 'Cakes are made mostly of starch and sugar that give you lots of energy' as being incorrect, he is marked wrong. The ignorruption around sugar and refined carbohydrates runs very deep indeed.

There is virtually no example in nature of the delivery of raw or 'empty' carbohydrates to any living creature. It is only the ingenuity of people, desperate to feed large volumes of consumers with cheap and long-shelf-life rubbish that has started to manipulate food in this way and convert it into junk.

We talk often in our society about 'junk food'. But 'junk food' is a poor description because it is not food at all. It should not be called food, it should not be sold as food and it should not be eaten as food.

Sugar is a toxic, addictive drug. It destroys our digestion, messes up our body's control systems, makes us fat and deprives our energy production plants of the essential nutrition they absolutely need to process energy.

Getting more energy, beneficially

So, back to our little furnaces. Think about them for a moment, little powerhouses, brilliantly able to convert real food into energy without any effort from you. If you nourish them well they will provide surpluses that can be put to good use.

And you can increase the number and output of these powerhouses simply by asking them to produce more. They will work harder, become more efficient and reproduce themselves to meet your demands. But, if you don't ask them to give you more energy then they will shrink, become tired and reduce in number.

It's all about energy: energy is life and the ultimate lack of energy is death. That's why any diet that implies that all calories are equal will kill you.

So, do you speak the language of your powerhouses? How can you ask them to give you more energy? Well, there is a way and it is very simple. But you have to really mean it. Because your powerhouses are smart, they will give you as much energy as you need but they won't give you any more than you need. People with low energy have low energy because the powerhouses are either running out of nutrients so their output reduces, or the energy that is produced is being used up desperately trying to get things back in balance. The amazing thing about your body is that no matter what happens it is always trying to heal itself, to be the best it can be, to do the best for you that it can.

So where is the energy switch? What do you have to do – pick up a loud hailer, point at your body and shout 'GIVE ME MORE ENERGY!'?

No, you need to be much more explicit than that. Your body is very intelligent but language only works with the conscious mind. The real intelligence of your body is that it responds to what is going on. It doesn't understand about 'food groups' that have been invented to sell products or 'calories' that come with no nutrition. Your body responds only to action. If you want energy you need to take action. Then the cells respond.

There is no short cut for this, I'm afraid. The only way to show your cells what you want is to show them what you want. Trying to tell them in words, wishing hard while you watch TV, sending messages while you read this book won't work of course. You have to take action.

The solution is: good quality fuel for good quality energy.

The action is only to supply fuel that comes with the nourishment needed to produce energy. No empty fuels. Any calorie that has been stripped of nourishment is an anti-energy calorie and it has a net negative effect. As soon as you add refined sugar or a refined grain to any food, you deplete its nutrient profile and it is always less healthy.

In the twenty-first century we eat foods that are predominantly anti-energy yet the helpful labels on the sides of the packet tell us how much 'energy' they contain. Ignorruption.

Only our conscious minds can process the language of the labels, the advertisements and the experts. The body understands the difference but we choose to believe the labels and the advertising, the nutrition 'experts' and the ignorrupt government ministers. The body tries hard to tell us. We eat the refined junk and the body goes into shock, after the momentary illusion of pleasure while it's in the mouth and the transient illusion of well-being as the sugar floods our blood. Then we sink to an energy low, craving another hit. Our bodies show us by dumping the rubbish as fat on our bellies, bottoms, upper legs, backs, upper arms: in

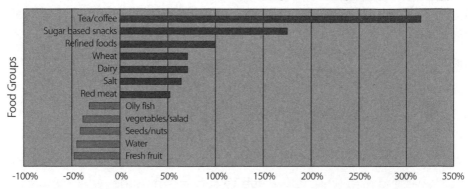

Food Group Consumption and Energy

This table shows the increase (dark grey) or reduction (light grey) in the likelihood of a very poor health score when comparing the consumption of various food groups.

obvious places to make us see it. It is a message from our body to stop. Yet we carry on.

Why do we carry on? Because our bodies crave nourishment. The body needs fuel. It cannot survive without it. The only way to get fuel is by eating nourishing foods. The more our nourishment is depleted by the junk the more our cravings increase. And then, sometimes we go on a diet. A 'calorie controlled diet' – but we don't change the profile of what we eat. The amount of junk we eat decreases, still with its anti-nutrient, anti-energy ingredients, but it is still there, even if in smaller quantities. And so our nourishment decreases and our cravings increase but we persist. We go to weekly group sessions where we are weighed and given points and calories and portions to count. We resist, we use willpower, we try really hard and, sure enough, some weight starts to come off. Depending on our levels of motivation, this can be kept up until the target on the scale is reached, but then we relax and go back to normal.

Metabolism

Our bodies don't understand the self-imposed restriction of food intake. They assume that we have gone into a famine and they start to shut down the metabolic process. Anything that can be put off is put off until another day when nourishment is more plentiful. And so the metabolism is slowed down and when the junk starts coming back in the whole process begins again. This time with the new fat slightly more flaccid, a little more sticky and a little more permanent.

I have women that come into my office who have been doing this for years. They do it when they are teenagers and they are still doing it when they are sixty. It is no way to live a life. Yet when they actually learn that not all calories are equal, that not all 'energy' is the same 'energy', then it becomes much easier for them to make changes.

It is utterly pointless to go on a 'calorie controlled diet' without adjusting the type of calories you eat. The cravings for junk come because you are malnourished and out of balance. To get rid of the cravings you need to be nourished and balanced – then vitality and well-being will come as if by magic.

Most people know that 100 calories of fresh, raw organic broccoli delivers more nourishment than 100 calories of refined sugar and this is the key. Here is a comparison of the nutrient profile of broccoli compared with white, refined sugar based on exactly the same calories:

Nutrient	Broccoli	Sugar	Extra nutrients in broccoli compared with sugar
Calories	100	100	
Carbohydrate	5.5	26.6	-389 per cent
Fat	2.7	0.0	100 per cent
Protein	13.3	0.0	100 per cent
Fibre	7.0	0.0	100 per cent
Minerals			
Sodium	24.2	0.0	100 per cent
Potassium	1121.2	0.5	100 per cent
Calcium	169.7	0.5	100 per cent
Magnesium	66.7	0.0	100 per cent
Phosphorous	263.6	0.0	100 per cent
Iron	5.2	0.0	100 per cent
Zinc	1.8	0.1	97 per cent
Manganese	0.6	0.0	100 per cent
Vitamins			
Carotene	1742.4	0.0	100 per cent
Thiamin	0.3	0.0	100 per cent
Riboflavin	0.2	0.0	100 per cent
Niacin	2.7	0.0	100 per cent
Vit B6	0.4	0.0	100 per cent
Folate	272.7	0.0	100 per cent
Vit C	263.6	0.0	100 per cent

It is knowing what this profile looks like that made my children laugh when the government minister suggested that we weren't getting fat because of the number of calories that we eat. Take a look at the nutritional profile, the nourishment profile of the calories we are eating. Of course the food lobbies want us to believe we are sick and fat because we don't exercise and only because we don't exercise. Heaven forbid that any sensible advice be given about reducing the intake of junk!

Unfortunately, on top of all this, the picture for broccoli isn't what it used to be. The mineral and vitamin contents of our vegetables has fallen by up to 75 per cent over the last 50 years, because of intensive farming techniques, low quality soils, the use of chemical fertilisers and the length of time it spends in transit. Gone are the days of good fresh vegetables from a local organic grower bought direct from your local greengrocer.

But back to the example. The broccoli, by anyone's measure, contains a lot of vitamins and minerals; the sugar contains none. The broccoli contains essential fibre that helps keep it moving through the digestive system; the sugar contains none. The broccoli contains protein, essential for the nourishment and growth of tissues and cells; the sugar contains none. The broccoli brings tiny quantities of natural fat that is useful to our cells

And this comparison does not take into consideration the other living nourishment that the broccoli brings with it.

Breathe, a nice deep breath. Who did you inhale atoms from this time?

Energy, living energy. The broccoli brings a host of living nutrients that we are only just beginning to learn about. They help protect the immune system, they provide enzymes to help the liver with detoxification. They have a living 'resonance' that energizes. The sugar has none of this. It is lifeless, dead, flat. It has nothing to offer.

To further press home the point let's imagine we are now preparing a TV ad and a label for our product SUGAR (as if we were an advertising agency acting on behalf of a sugar peddler) and we want to gain a commercial advantage over our competitor BROCCOLI.

What could we say? We could say:

SUGAR – 100 PER CENT LESS FAT THAN BROCCOLI!
No need to mention that the fats in broccoli are pure, natural essential fats that are useful to the body

SUGAR – 100 PER CENT FAT FREE!
No need to mention that while the sugar contains no fat in the packet it will almost certainly turn straight to fat in your body, as your pancreas is forced to spurt insulin into your bloodstream to eliminate the excess sugar. And no need to mention that the stress that this places on your pancreas might undermine your body's response to insulin, or even wear out your body's ability to make insulin, so that you end up diabetic.

SUGAR – PURE ENERGY!
Calories are energy, right? No need to mention it doesn't bring any of the nutrients required to process them and it will therefore have to suck nutrients out of your body, so robbing you of energy.

SUGAR – RICH IN VITAMIN C! MADE WITH REAL JUICE!
Just so we can make the claim we'll add a bit of Vitamin C to it. Mothers think that Vitamin C is good for children and they will buy things that are 'rich' in vitamins. We could add to the scam by adding a bit of concentrated, pasteurised blackcurrant juice (for example) – this will give it an appealing colour so kids will like it and then we could improve our claim…

It is everywhere. Labels are utterly mislead.
to give you any nourishment information at all.
panel on the average label tells us little of any w
the dark.

But your cells know the difference. They can fe
energy that come from clean, living foods. So do them......ow them
you need energy and take action to deliver them foods that show them
you want energy. Complete lack of energy is death. Complete abundance
of energy is life, total vitality, complete well-being. Anything in the middle is
a compromise. Any refined food is a compromise. It will 'unbalance' your
diet and compromise your health. Remember we mentioned earlier that
the 'healthy balanced diet' was being discarded in favour of the 'healthy
varied diet'. It's because you can't really escape the maths. And so the
corporate institutions that educate us about nutrition want us to believe
that variety is what we're after to be healthy. Because, after 50 years of the
notion of 'balance', people have started to do the maths.

My six-year-old can work out that broccoli contains more nourishment
than sugar and she knows what sugar does. I haven't told her that broccoli
is 'good' and sugar is 'bad', just what happens inside her body when she
eats them. One is food the other is not food. It's important to know the
difference: that one contains helpful, beneficial nourishment that makes
her cells happy and healthy; that the other contains nothing except an
illusion of taste, an illusion of energy, that can interfere with her digestion,
rob her cells of energy and increase her chances dramatically of ending up
dying from an unnecessary, degenerative disease.

Is she banned from eating junk? By no means. She is living in a world
where this rubbish is on sale at virtually every retail outlet. The newsagent,
the garage, the supermarket, the leisure centre, her ballet class. It is
everywhere. There is no escape for her or for you. Proper nourishment has

...me down to knowledge, understanding, self-reliance and self-reference. The government ministers will continue to be hoodwinked by the corporate PR consultants and food industry lobbies for a long time yet. Sugar is a dangerous drug. It kills. Be aware. Be careful.

The route to obesity, heart disease, diabetes and cancer

Eating 'food' that does not nourish leaves the body starving	**Eat 'food' that is contaminated and/or depleted**	Tinned 'foods', Processed 'foods', Refined 'foods', Restaurant 'foods', Instant 'foods'
No amount of junk can nourish the body. It craves real nutrition	**Crave more food. Feel hungry**	Interference with palate and poor quality 'food' messes up our hunger signals
Not knowing the difference between junk and food makes for bad decisions	**Eat 'food' that is contaminated and/or depleted**	Interference with palate and poor quality 'food' messes up our hunger signals
The body becomes clogged, malnourished, fat and unwell	**Feel tired and lethargic**	Lack of nourishment leads to lack of energy (in spite of all the calories eaten)
Evolutionary cravings for sweet, fat and salt are misinterpreted and more junk is consumed	**Crave sugar and refined foods**	Increasing cravings for junk – confectionery, sodas, tea, coffee, cakes and refined 'food'
Refined 'foods' set up hormonal and metabolic swings that wear out vital organs and create an energy 'roller coaster'	**After brief 'high' a slump then leads to need for another 'hit'**	Continued cravings or preferences for sweet, salty and fatty 'foods'
Cycle can be partially mitigated against by eating fruit, vegetables, drinking water, exercising and taking supplementation. These can all help but do not offer immunity from the effects of junk.	**OBESITY, DISEASE, HEART DISEASE, MENTAL DISORDERS, CANCER AND PREMATURE DEATH**	The only real solution is the removal of junk from your food intake. Sugar, refined grains, stimulants, pesticides, hormones, contaminated meat and dairy included.

Because the solution is commercially and politically unacceptable it is down to you, the individual, to take personal action. The labels, advertisements and ingredients will, eventually, change but it won't be in time to help your decisions or your life.

Back to our cells; how best to give them clean, nourishing fuel for energy? The first way we have discussed is by feeding them foods that deliver living energy and nourishment. Raw or lightly cooked vegetables; beans, sprouted or cooked; legumes; whole grains; living foods, these are the foods that will nourish your cells. They bring with them the vitamins, minerals, enzymes, plant nutrients, fibre and overall nourishment that will fire your furnaces. This is step one in your call for your cells to produce energy.

Breathing life into our cells

The only way to get enough oxygen to your cells is by breathing; deep, regular breathing. Try it now. Take ten long deep breaths. Inhale right to the bottom of your lungs, really try to get as much air in as you possibly can. When you think your lungs are full, suck in a bit more, and a bit more. Good. Hold each one for a few seconds and then exhale slowly.

Take the ten breaths now.

Did you do it?

Yes? Great. You're telling your cells you want energy and you're prepared to give them what they need. Notice the difference in your body from taking the deep breaths. You can feel it. Notice the energization taking place – take a deep breath and notice how long it takes to feel the difference it makes in your feet.

Taking in oxygen is critical. So we're going to start talking to our cells with action; eating living, nourishing foods and breathing fully. But I said something about moving. What did I mean?

Well, movement is the most direct call for energy that you can make.

Stand up in a moment. Stand up straight and well balanced. Head up, pulled upright by an imaginary thread that tugs at the top of your head. Relax your shoulders fully and lift your arms up to the side keeping them straight. Then circle your hands 25 times forwards and 25 times backwards. Breathe deeply the whole time.

Go ahead and do it.

Welcome back.

Notice the feeling in your shoulders. That is your cells working. They have been producing energy to enable those little arm rotations. Many people feel a 'burn' in their shoulders when they do this because if our cells aren't used to being called on to produce energy, they do it inefficiently and can produce waste products that cause the 'burn'. Some people used to think that getting this 'burn' was necessary to improve strength and energy but it is not.

Get moving

Movement is the most direct call for energy that you can make of your cells. To move you have to produce energy, to move a lot you have to produce a lot of energy. So a gradually increasing amount of movement is what you're after. This doesn't mean rushing out to a health club and doing a hamster impersonation on a treadmill. This kind of mindless exercise is boring and repetitive and far less effective both mentally and physically than more natural movement. But the health club can, in fact, play a part, and this is how I suggest you use it. These days you can usually find a health club within a mile or two of your home or place of work. Find out where it is and walk to it. Walk briskly but not so you get out of breath. When you get there, look in through the window at the people running on the treadmill and then look at all the cars parked in the car park. Then laugh to yourself and walk briskly back home.

Do this every day for the next 30 days. It will cost you nothing and you will grow in energy. Your cells will start to realize that you want them to produce energy and, if you feed them well, they will produce it efficiently. You will find, day by day, that you can walk more briskly without getting out of breath. This is important, the not-getting-out-of-breath bit. The best way to produce energy is in the presence of oxygen. If you have to gasp when you start to get out of breath, this is a signal that you are exceeding your oxygen energy capacity. Slow down and get back into a comfortable rhythm. It's fine to breathe deeply and feel your heart working, that is what movement needs. But don't push too hard. And so, very simple things can make a huge difference: walking the children to school or walking to work, or parking the car a mile or so away and then walking; parking at the farthest end of the supermarket car park and carrying your bags instead of wheeling them in a trolley; carrying a basket around the supermarket rather than wheeling a trolley. You'll buy less and create more energy!

It's pretty obvious really.

Listen to your body

Eat foods that give real energy. Call for more energy directly from your cells by moving more. Your cells will grow their energy production capacity; your metabolic rate will rise; your furnaces will start to burn more brightly; your digestion will become more efficient; you will get more from your food; your cells will create more energy; you will feel an urge to move more, to eat better, to feel more energetic – another wonderful positive spiral.

As your furnaces burn more brightly your body will begin to normalize. Your liver will be able to filter and process more thoroughly and efficiently. As your cells get fitter and more efficient they will generate more little powerhouses and create more energy. Balance will begin to be restored.

Incidentally, in many cultures, people are strongly discouraged from eating the leftovers from cooked meals. Leftovers from cooked meals tend to be lifeless, flat and heavy and are hard to digest, yet, in our age of convenience, we buy 'pre-prepared' meals. They come in foil cartons with cardboard tops that show pictures of food that make you salivate in anticipation. All you have to do is heat them up.

Eating ready meals is the same as eating leftovers. These are not foods – they are junk. Junk is now in every category and area of the food industry.

Be your own expert. Do your own maths. Notice how you feel. Look at the diagram below and think of your goal. Remember what perfection will look and feel like. Then make decisions and take action.

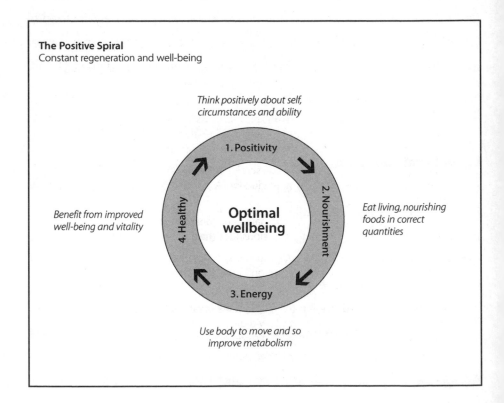

The Positive Spiral
Constant regeneration and well-being

Think positively about self, circumstances and ability

1. Positivity

2. Nourishment

Eat living, nourishing foods in correct quantities

Optimal wellbeing

4. Healthy

Benefit from improved well-being and vitality

3. Energy

Use body to move and so improve metabolism

Give yourself the gift of energetic cells and a glowing metabolism

Objective:
To enable your cells to produce abundant energy, efficiently and cleanly with a minimum of waste and to allow this energy to fire up your digestion and all body systems so your body operates in balance and harmony.

Benefits:
Your body will normalize fat storage and become leaner. Skin condition will improve. Your mind will be clearer and you will feel much more positive and in control. You will be able to do more and cope with more. You will be healthier with a better immune system. Your bones and muscles will be stronger.

Strategies:
1. Eat fruit. Whole, fresh fruits. As wide a variety as you can. They contain natural sugars in the presence of living plant nutrients, enzymes, vitamins and minerals. Living energy.

2. Eat vegetables. Green leafy vegetables and brightly coloured vegetables. Vegetables, like fruits, are power-packed sources of living energy that come with all the nutrients needed to convert them to energy.

3. Eat whole foods. Eat grains and legumes that are complete. Brown rice, whole wheat, beans and lentils. They provide carbohydrates along with vitamins, minerals, oils, enzymes and proteins.

4. Breathe deeply. Do this consciously every day. Deep breathing while you focus on inhaling fully and exhaling completely.

5. Move. Walk, play, run, jump, cycle, swim, play some more. Get your heart rate up and your breathing increased but do not get out of breath. Move as much as you can and, at least once a day, get up and move deliberately, just for the sake of moving.

6. Eat nuts and seeds. Fresh raw nuts and seeds contain essential oils and loads of minerals that are crucial to energy production. A fantastic boost to your nourishing food intake.

7. Avoid refined foods. Minimize or eliminate your consumption of refined sugar and white flour. Read labels and look consciously for the addition of drugs like sugar.

8. Avoid stimulants. Coffee and tea are drugs that give an illusion of energy but that compromise digestion and liver function. Replace with fresh juices and hot fruit toddies.

9. Minimize your consumption of animal products. Meat and dairy products place large demands on digestive energy and slow digestion. Eat animal products in extremely small quantities, certainly not daily and never at more than one meal a day.

SKIN – OUR FIRST LINE OF DEFENCE

There is an old saying that 'beauty comes from within'. There is huge emphasis in our fashion-conscious world on the quality and youthfulness of skin. It goes along with largely irrational, enforced and transient views about what size we should be, how large or small women's breasts should be, and what is 'youthful' or 'attractive'.

The condition of skin is held up as an icon of beauty. Fortunes are spent on lotions and potions that promise rejuvenation, removal of wrinkles, moisturizing qualities, nutrition… the list is endless.

Cleanse. Tone. Moisturize. A daily routine for many on the quest for youthful, great-looking skin.

But there is a lot more to skin than meets the eye. Healthy skin has a vital role to play in your overall well-being. But does healthy skin come from within? Or do you need to rub stuff on it to keep it in shape?

The skin is the largest organ in the human body. As such, it performs a number of critical functions that connect it intimately with all your important body systems. There is a direct correlation between 'beauty' and skin, particularly in western culture. The majority of western media is filled with images of people, generally women, with apparently perfect skin. For the most part, this perfection is an illusion. It is usual for the face of a photographic model to be caked with over 1mm of makeup to ensure that any underlying skin blemishes are hidden and to assist the proper absorption and reflection of light for the camera.

'Good' skin is much prized, particularly by women, and skin complaints, especially those that affect the face, are the cause of enormous anguish and stress to people.

So, to what extent does beautiful skin reflect a beautiful body inside? If the skin is suffering we can see it dry, flaky, spotty, oily, stretched or wrinkly.

The equivalent problems with brains, hearts, livers, kidneys, glands, bones or muscles are not so readily identified. In this respect, skin can be quite a good motivator once we become aware that it is operating with the rest of our body to try and help everything remain in balance.

The outer layer of skin is made up of flat cells that resemble paving stones. Its thickness varies, depending on the part of the body. It is thickest on the soles of your feet and the palms of your hands. It is very thin on the eyelids. It is generally thicker in men than in women and has a tendency to become thinner as you grow older.

The outermost part of the skin is made up of dead cells, which form a protective coating. As these dead cells are worn away, they are replaced. The new cells are produced by rapidly dividing living cells in the innermost part of the outer layer.

Most of the cells in the outer layer are specialized to produce keratin, a hard protein substance that is the main constituent of the tough, outermost part. Some of the cells produce the protective pigment melanin, which determines skin colour.

A deeper layer of skin is made up of connective tissue which contains various specialized structures, such as hair follicles, sweat glands, and sebaceous glands (glands that produce an oily substance called 'sebum'). This layer also contains blood vessels, lymph vessels (that carry waste), and nerves (that carry sensory information).

Your skin is intimately connected to your body in its entirety, both literally and metaphorically. It has some very important functions.

Nature's armour

Your skin's most important function is a protective one. It acts as a barrier between your environment and the internal organs of your body. The skin shields your body from injury, the harmful rays of sunlight, and invasion

> *Rehydration – the simplicity of water – goes a long way towards banishing wrinkles*

from infective agents, such as bacteria and viruses.

Your skin is a sensitive organ. It contains millions of cells that are sensitive to touch, temperature, vibration, pain, pressure, and itching. By using these cells it warns you when to move away from dangerous situations – when something is too hot, too sharp, too irritating or too heavy.

Your skin also plays an important role in keeping body temperature constant. When the body is hot your sweat glands cool it by producing perspiration and the blood vessels in the skin are able to widen to get rid of excess heat. If your body gets cold, the blood vessels in the skin can squeeze themselves narrower to conserve your body's heat. It is important to exercise these sweat glands and keep your skin exercised, to ensure the efficient working of this system. You can do this by engaging in movement that raises your body temperature to the point that you raise a gentle sweat or glow. Doing this by exercise is more effective than by using a sauna or steam room because it gets the blood flowing in the lower layers of your skin. This promotes skin growth and regeneration and maintains effective fluid balance in the skin.

The outer layer of your skin contains a unique fatty substance that makes the skin waterproof. You should be very thankful for this one-way waterproofing. If it wasn't there and you sat in a bath you would soak water up like a sponge until you were about 20 times your normal size. This outer layer also has an effective water-holding capacity, which helps to keep it flexible. It has the duty also of helping to keep your body in fluid and electrolyte balance. If the water content of skin drops below a certain level, the skin becomes cracked, reducing its efficiency as a barrier. You should avoid interfering with this outer layer by clogging it up with creams and oils. You need to make sure you consume essential fatty acids to keep the fatty layer intact. This will keep your skin elastic and flexible. To keep your skin moist and your skin cells plump and hydrated, the only effective means is to drink fresh water, at least seven to eight glasses a day. No, rubbing water on your skin does NOT work; moisturizing can only be done effectively by water via the mouth! A useful example of how this works is to remember that if you or someone you know has cracked lips, try this: drink a glass of fresh water. Drink another one 20–30 minutes later. Keep going. Within two hours the cracking will start to disappear as water reaches your dehydrated cells.

Another of your skin's most critical functions is as an organ of elimination. It helps your body get rid of waste. Apart from excess heat, the skin also serves as an 'overflow' channel of elimination for the rest of the body. The body is capable of depositing excess toxic materials in the outer layer of the skin. This is fine if it is in small quantities, but excess toxicity combined with dehydration and inadequate vitamins and minerals can cause skin problems. Maintaining good circulation in the skin and encouraging the removal of the dead cells from the surface is the best way to ensure the skin keeps effectively regenerating. Brushing with a gentle bristle brush before your morning shower is a fabulous way to encourage circulation, dead cell removal and skin regeneration. Many people think that this will make skin tough and hard – exactly the opposite is true – it becomes silky soft and smooth.

Another way of 'exercising' the circulation in your skin is to use hot and cold showers. You can do this at the end of your daily shower by running the water as hot as you can stand it for 30–60 seconds; then run it as cold as you can stand it for 30 seconds or so. Repeat this three to five times, ending on cold. This stimulates the circulation in your skin and pumps blood in and out of the lower layers with the blood vessels getting narrower and then wider. It is fabulous for your skin's health.

Is beauty, indeed, only skin deep?

Does 'beautiful' skin reflect a healthy body? The answer is that it can do but not always. There are a lot of things you can do, though, to help keep your skin in great shape so it can help you keep in balance. Also a lot of things you can do to help keep excessive demands off your skin.

Skin needs to be well nourished. Now, let's get something clear about nourishing skin. What is the best way to get nutrients to your skin? Consider this:

Nature designed my body with a brilliantly designed digestive system, 60,000 miles of blood vessels and 75 trillion cells with their own perfect nutrient supply system and waste disposal mechanism so that I could feed it most effectively by rubbing cream on it.

True or false?

I know you will find this difficult to accept, but there are a great many people who hold the belief that they can effectively cleanse, nourish and hydrate their skin by rubbing cream on it.

Extraordinary I know, but there are still a lot of people who are very ignorant about how their skin works and this is compounded by watching too many TV commercials. In these advertisements, messages from 'beautiful' celebrities and announcements from big international companies with a great many patents, have finally convinced them there is some merit in the cream-rubbing phenomenon.

What is the best way to hydrate your skin?

What is the best way to protect your skin?

What is the best way to rejuvenate your skin?

What is the best way to get rid of wrinkles?

If you don't know already you're about to find out. But you can rest assured it does not involve skin creams, lotions or potions. Creams sell an illusion, a dream, a wish for result without change.

Next time you pick up a fashion magazine take it with you to a public swimming pool on a Sunday afternoon. Look at the pictures of the people in the magazine and then look at the people in the pool. Hold them up, one eye on the magazine and one eye on the pool. Observe the illusion and the reality.

Now decide which is your reality. What do people look like? How do you feel when you compare the reality of your body, your looks, with the people in the magazine? How do you feel when you compare the reality of your body, your looks, with the people in the pool? In fact neither is relevant to you. Because you are your own perfect reality.

How perfect are you? Utterly!

But back to your skin. We've discussed how it is structured and what it does. Constantly growing and regenerating, it breeds itself in lower levels, has a section made up of live and dead cells that can allow gases and fluids out and prevent fluids coming in. On the outside there is a protective layer of dead cells that flake off constantly. In this way skin helps with the elimination of waste, provides protection, helps with temperature control, the balance of body fluids, and keeps everything hanging together.

Feed your skin – from the inside

First let's consider the nutrition of the skin. Skin relies on plenty of vitamin C to form collagen. If vitamin C is deficient then collagen production is impaired. Collagen is an elastic substance that gives your skin flexibility along with a substance called elastin. Both collagen and elastin can be damaged by free radicals. Free radicals are scavenging molecules that are produced as by-products of the body's metabolism. They are also formed by the combustion of bad foods (particularly bad fats) and from overcooked and burned foods.

The skin, along with your whole body, needs access to antioxidants to protect itself from free radicals. Vitamins A, C and E and the minerals selenium and zinc are required to provide the skin with this protection. There are a hundred creams that promise to deliver these vitamins and minerals by rubbing them on. But the skin is designed to resist the entry of foreign substances. To try and nourish it this way is absolutely futile.

The only really effective way to get protective antioxidants to the skin is via the fabulous network of blood vessels that run through its lower layers. It is quite pointless to try to nourish the dead cells on the surface because they are about to be discarded. Skin cream is one of the most futile and ridiculous scams ever thought of. But it is proof that ignorruption works. Like the story of the emperor's new clothes, people will continue to say they can see the clothes even though they are clearly confronted by the king's nudity.

Vitamin A (best obtained as beta carotene) is required to limit production of a substance called keratin in the outer layer of the skin. Excess keratin can result in dry, rough skin and Vitamin A can help ensure this does not take place. Cell membranes, our skin cells included, are made from essential fats. A lack of essential fats can allow skin to dry out too quickly resulting in dryness and cracking. Also, the presence of damaged and unnatural fats can compromise skin condition. Avoid eating hydrogenated fats, any foods containing trans-fats and say 'no' to heated vegetable oils (often used for frying).

Supplementation is a particularly good way of caring for your skin

Skin health depends on adequate zinc, which is needed for accurate reproduction of all cells. Zinc deficiency can lead to stretch marks or poor healing.

These nutrients are all critical not just to the skin

but, as we know, they are needed by other body systems. The antioxidants are required to protect all cells from free radical damage and they play an important role in the immune system. Essential fats are critical for cardiovascular health, for the immune system, for the endocrine and nervous systems.

So we can see that dry or rough skin, stretch marks, tight, wrinkly skin can all represent nutritional disorders that may reflect underlying problems in other body systems. The difference is that, because the skin is on the outside, we can see it. The effects are more obvious. In this respect the skin can act as a window on the body, and skin disorders that reflect nutritional deficiency probably indicate underlying health problems.

External factors

Other skin problems can result from external influences such as exposure to chemicals or the sun. Reactions to these sorts of influences vary markedly between individuals and the underlying health of the body will, of course, influence the reaction or response. A powerful immune system will reduce the likelihood of dermatitis, for example, and plenty of anti-inflammatory prostaglandins (due to adequate essential fatty acids and effective EFA metabolism) will reduce chances of allergic reactions to external influences or indeed food.

So, skin problems such as dermatitis or eczema are likely to reflect underlying immune and digestive imbalances more than they reflect the health of the skin itself.

Cellulite and oily skin can reflect excess body loads of saturated or damaged fats and a toxic burden that the body is trying to keep somewhere 'safe' until it can be eliminated. These skin conditions can, therefore, reflect the collection of morbid matter in the system that can cause problems in other body systems. The effect of excess saturated fat in the cardiovascular system is well known and any build-up of unwanted toxins has potentially disastrous consequences for health.

Can an unhealthy body have good skin?

It is largely true that skin problems reflect underlying health problems. It is worth recognizing though that when a body has the energy to detoxify after a period of intake and collection of toxic waste, there can be a reaction in skin as some of the toxins are released through the skin; in perspiration, for example. In some circles these skin reactions are seen as part of a 'healing crisis' and reflect a gradual improvement in body condition.

'Good' skin can however mask very deep-lying disease conditions. Many people have skin problems that 'disappear' after a time. Children that present eczema in early years often find it disappears later in life. Many adolescent skin complaints disappear, with the catch-all 'it must have been their hormones' being used to explain the improvement in skin condition.

The skin, it is said, can hide an underlying toxic state because the body simply doesn't have the resources or energy to produce a skin reaction. It is well known for cancer victims who follow natural regimes for cure to get progressively worse skin conditions as healing progresses. They come in with good skin when they're dying and leave with apparently poorer skin when they're healing. It's all part of the ebb and flow of body balances.

So one has to be careful of jumping to conclusions about the message that a skin complaint is giving. Yes, it probably represents an underlying imbalance but it is important to discover in which direction the individual is headed. It is always worth supporting your overall health with nutritional supplementation if you have poor skin.

To obtain and keep fantastic, healthy skin here's what to do:

Give yourself the gift of fabulous, beautiful, effective skin

Objective:
To keep skin flexible, strong, smooth and healthy and help it execute its essential functions of protection, control, regeneration and elimination.

Benefits:
Skin that stays young longer, fewer wrinkles, better skin colour and smooth, silky-feeling skin.

Strategies:

1. Get your body to a gentle sweat for 30 minutes at least three times a week. Do this by moving and exercising rather than by a sauna or steam room. This stimulates blood supply and lymphatic drainage.

2. Stimulate skin regeneration and elimination of dead surface cells by brushing with a soft to medium bristle brush before you shower or bathe. Do this every day or at least 3 times a week.

3. Stimulate the blood supply to your lower skin layers by alternating hot and cold 3–5 times each day at the end of your morning shower.

4. Ensure you get plenty of vitamin C in your diet. In addition to vitamin C-rich foods, take at least 1 gram of vitamin C a day.

5. Eat foods rich in the antioxidant vitamins A and E. In particular, ensure you are getting enough Vitamin A. The antioxidant minerals zinc and selenium are also important.

6. Ensure your essential fatty acid intake is adequate. The best way to get them is by occasionally eating oily fish and by taking a tablespoon of a good organic oil blend each day as well as a handful of fresh raw nuts and seeds.

7. Avoid foods that contribute to free radical activity. These include overcooked and burned foods, unnatural fats and heated vegetable oils. These damaged fats can find their way into your skin's cell membranes and affect skin condition.

8. Drink plenty of fresh water. This is essential to keep skin cells plump and hydrated. The only effective way to moisturize!

9. Avoid skin creams and oils as far as possible. It may take a bit of time to wean yourself away but it is worth pursuing.

10. Avoid the use of soap on your skin. This will diminish your perceived need for skin cream.

IMMUNITY – YOUR NATURAL BARRIERS AND DEFENCES

Our natural lifespan is thought to be about 120 years. But few of us make it that far. Most of us will die well before we are 80 with an unnecessary, debilitating degenerative disease. It is likely to be diabetes, heart disease or cancer along with a number of other painful or inconvenient conditions including arthritis, osteoporosis, incontinence, depression and memory loss.

Not a great prognosis. This is surprising to many people who think that we have made great strides over the last century in improving and optimizing lifespan. But this simply isn't true. Age-adjusted statistics show that the lifespan of a healthy man or woman has not moved much in 100 years. And in any event most of the advances that have been made are due to sanitation, better housing, less war and safer workplaces.

We have got much better, it has to be said, at keeping people with diseases alive for longer. And this is the focus of modern medicine. The ambulances and health centres are built at the bottom of the cliff to repair people who fall over it. And most of us do.

So we can expect to live, incapacitated with heart disease for a few years more. Many will live for many years, injecting themselves with insulin or other drugs. Some will live a few more years permanently mutilated by aggressive surgical procedures, vicious drug treatments or burning (radiation) to treat cancers.

Yet it is perfectly possible to live to 100 or beyond in excellent health with all faculties intact and to die, when ready, peacefully in your sleep having held your great-grandchildren in your arms.

Have you chosen what you're going to die of? What? You didn't think you had a choice?

Malnourished? Yes, you are

Luck? Your genes? Your environment? Who or what do you think decides your destiny?

The answer is that all of the above may play a role and none of us is in complete control. But we do have a lot of control and it is our choice whether to exercise it or not.

Studies on healthy centenarians carried out over the last few years have shown one particularly noticeable trait that is not present in less well peers. The healthy old-timers have excellent immune systems.

The major reason for weakened immune system function is depletion of the nutrients that the immune system needs to work effectively. It is possible to dramatically improve immune system function at any age by supplying the body with the nutrients it needs.

Could it really be that we are dying early because of malnutrition? With all the incredible progress we have made with modern medicine, could it possibly be as simple as being malnourished?

Well, I'm afraid so.

Take almost any official statistics in any Western nation and you'll find that vitamin and mineral depletion is rampant. Even compared with the RDAs (Recommended Daily Allowances) we are depleted, and these RDAs were only ever set to avoid known deficiency diseases. They are at least 50 years out of date and were never designed on the basis of optimizing our health. If we ran an analysis of nutrition today using any sensible programme of research we would take the nutrient intake of Western populations and work out that what we were eating was causing heart disease, diabetes and cancer. Then we could compare that with the diet of groups of people who live to 100 or more in good health.

These studies have been done and, surprise surprise, the individuals who live longer get more nourishment in their meals, live less stressful lives and are more active. It isn't rocket science.

Immunity is a 'choice' issue

However, it is important to note that the 'lower' down the lifestyle scale people are, the more likely it is that they will be malnourished and deficient in key nutrients. These deficiencies set up a series of negative spirals including those we've already discussed: declining digestive efficiency, adverse liver function, blood sugar swings and fat deposition and low energy. A natural consequence of this negative cascade is a depleted immune system.

Your immune system is your internal police force. It is a second line of defence. Your first lines of defence begins with skin that keeps things out, your digestive system which tries to keep invaders out and your liver that screens for terrorists. But your body and your blood is a swirling cocktail of micro-organisms. Bacteria, viruses, parasites, yeasts all have the potential for getting in and causing trouble. These things are all in your body now and your immune system is dealing with them. There is no escape. Our immune system has a series of specialist cells that are designed to seek out and destroy any of these unwanted organisms that cause trouble.

It is thought that cancers start to grow relatively frequently in our bodies. They don't, for the most part, become a problem because the immune system spots the cells that have gone awry and despatches killer cells to nip them in the bud.

Some people believe that they can 'catch' a cold. The germ theory of disease is very popular. But many studies show that the viruses or bacteria that are supposedly responsible for the cold or flu are often present in the bodies of people who do not present with the symptoms. In an epidemic of any disease there are always people who don't get it. Yet they have undoubtedly been exposed. Why is this?

It is the efficiency of the immune system that is key. Your immune defences need to be kept in tip-top condition. There are two key factors to consider when it comes to boosting your immunity. The first is getting enough of the immune–boosting nutrients and the second is living a life in which you are happy, relaxed and as free of stress as possible.

Key nutrients

Let's begin with the key nutrients: the essential vitamins and minerals necessary to keep your immune system strong and efficient.

Vitamin C might be termed the master immune vitamin. It has a wide range of roles in the maintenance and stimulation of immune response and effectiveness. Vitamin C in itself has antiviral properties and its presence can prevent or at least inhibit viral infection. An immune cell destruction system where foreign cells are surrounded, captured and killed is completely dependent on Vitamin C in adequate quantities.

Vitamin A is a powerful anti-viral vitamin that helps your cells to resist viral attack, by maintaining strong linings in areas prone to risk of infection; in particular, your nose, throat and lungs, your digestive system and your urinary tract. An antibacterial enzyme found in tears, saliva and sweat is dependent on Vitamin A for its production. This enzyme is also found in immune cells.

Calcium is required by immune cells to help them stick to foreign bodies. Fever production is calcium-dependent and running a fever is a great way to burn off unwanted organisms. We tend to be far too quick these days to suppress fevers and fewer and fewer people have the energy to run a good fever anymore.

Magnesium is needed to keep up antibody levels and to produce immune factors. Antibody production is dependent on iron. Zinc indirectly influences immune cell activity.

All of these nutrients are commonly depleted in most people. The RDAs of these are too low for optimization of immune function and even fresh foods simply do not contain these nutrients in the quantities they used to.

Our early ancestors probably ate a quantity of food that amounted to an equivalent of around 4,000 calories a day. All fresh, recently picked, organic food: predominantly fruit, vegetables, roots, nuts, seeds, grubs, a bit of fish and the occasional small animal. Not to mention the consistent, gentle exercise they were getting whilst gathering it! We now eat 2,000 or so calories a day of depleted junk that provides a fraction of the nutrients we need, and yet we still have the same physical bodies of our ancestors of thousands of years ago. The foodstuffs we were evolved to eat are more and more ignored as the myriad choices of today's food production have sent the relationship between our wants and our requirements haywire.

We can do a lot with sensible food choices but not enough, I'm afraid. It is essential to supplement your food intake with additional nutrients. High quality nutrients in sensible quantities in forms that it is easy for the body to absorb.

Many of my clients are shocked at the thought that they can't get what they need from their food. 'It's not natural', they say. They are right – it is not natural and it is not ideal – but it is a fact of life.

Driving a car instead of walking isn't natural. Eating foods that have been stripped of all their nutrition isn't natural. Eating the carcasses of animals that are riddled with pesticides, antibiotics and hormones isn't natural. Inhaling the toxic by-products of the combustion of petroleum spirit isn't natural. Eating food heated by irradiation with microwaves isn't natural. Taking chemical drugs to suppress the symptoms of our unnatural lives isn't natural.

Get real. Get some nutrients in addition to those you get from food.

A daily, high quality multinutrient is essential. It should contain the essential minerals and vitamins in significant amounts. Don't take the rubbish that is sold by the big brands that advertise on television. They do not contain useful forms of most of the minerals, and the quantities are so low as to be barely worthwhile. You would probably do better to suck on the cardboard boxes they come in.

Go to a decent health outlet and get a high quality multinutrient. There are many of them about. Switch brands often, say, every month. Each manufacturer has different forms and different amounts. Variety is a good idea with nutrients, as it is with your food.

Your immune system and your whole body will thank you for it.

Most of us will die of malnutrition. Bad food choices and inadequate intakes of key nutrients are the cause. There is legislation going through the EU at the time of writing that threatens to restrict your ability to buy nutritional supplements in adequate quantities. The legislation is positioned as being in your best interests from a safety and quality perspective but it is an ignorruption scam I'm afraid. It is designed to place the balance of power in favour of drug manufacturing interests and to prevent consumers from making effective health choices. There is far more evidence of the damaging effects of sugar, coffee, dairy products and meat than there is for nutritional supplements, but there is no attempt to legislate against these products. Why? Because it is all about money, ignorruption and the stupidity of government and legislators who are naïve, stupid, ignorant or corrupt, or a combination of all of these.

You have to look out for yourself, I'm afraid.

Stress and your immunity

I mentioned that your state of mind is important for your immune system. It is critical. Freedom from stress and anxiety is a key factor.

There are numerous examples of actors who have to play depressed, sad or stressed parts, and they become stricken themselves with ghastly diseases, until they are able to come out of character and once again restore their immunity. Your mind and your body are completely intertwined. We have already described the interconnection of your digestive system and your mind; remember the all-important 'gut feeling'? Well, so it is with your immune system.

You will have heard the expression 'laughter is your best medicine'. This isn't a flippant statement. Laughing at the idiots around you, laughing at yourself and laughing at the stupidity of it all has a lot to be said for it.

All it takes is five minutes...

Relax. Take a deep breath and allow your body to soften completely. Start with the little muscles at the side of your mouth. Do it now. Relax your eyes. Breathe. Think of a really comfortable place. Somewhere you feel warm and cosseted and safe. Picture yourself in this safe place. Breathe, and, as you breathe, notice how you are able to relax even further as you see yourself in total comfort and peace. It feels like being taken on a journey in your mind to a place where nothing can happen that doesn't make you feel strong, and where you hear kind voices saying pleasant things to you while you are bathed in comforting colours. Breathe. Notice the effect of your breathing and make a clear picture of your truly comfortable place. Turn up the colours and bring the picture closer. Hear the sounds you hear when you are completely relaxed and at peace, see the things you see and sense how the different parts of your body relax and feel softer as you breathe, and notice the beginnings of a new and improved immune system.

If you did what was asked, it is likely that in the last few seconds you actually created more immune power, just by relaxing and thinking pleasant thoughts.

Do it again. This time really focus on the comfort and relaxation. Take five minutes. Go on, it's only five minutes.

Welcome back.

Did you do it?

Yes: you're on the way. No: you're on a different path.

Remember, if you keep doing what you've always done you'll keep getting what you've always got. Take new paths, go to new places. Get out of your rut and open your mind, open your eyes, open your ears. Don't listen to me, listen to the world; look around you and investigate with interest; feel what things do to you and make sure you focus on the things that feel good, REALLY feel good. Watch out for the illusions and the pressures of custom, convention and social pressure.

Making intelligent decisions about what to eat does not usually make other people feel good. They need excuses and reinforcement to make their own decisions OK. And so the 'sensible' eater is derided for being 'faddy', 'goody two-shoes', 'on a diet'. Expect this and ride it. It will soon be forgotten. Occasionally accept the offering. You don't have to eat or drink it. But sometimes it's just easier to run with the situation and keep everyone else feeling comfortable. Whatever you do, don't try and lecture them about why you have changed. They will not thank you for it. If they ask why you've changed what you eat and drink, you can legitimately confirm that you are not on a diet and you never intend ever to go on another diet again. Tell them you've decided to 'Live it'.

Be calm and in control. It will give you an inner power that delivers all sorts of unexpected benefits. Eat nourishing foods, take a decent food supplement and relax.

What else affects your immunity?

Lymph system

It's time to talk about your largest circulation system: the lymph system. Now, unless you've done a bit of biology or physiology you may not know a lot about it. It is a series of tubes and channels, much like the circulation system your blood uses. But it doesn't have a pump. It relies on your movement and breathing to make its contents move. Your lymph system is the waste disposal system of your body. One of its main functions is to carry waste away from your cells and filters it before passing treated waste back into the bloodstream, where it can be dealt with by your liver and kidneys before it leaves your body in the form of faeces or urine.

Deliberate movement and moderate exercise are essential for an effective and efficient lymph system. But beware, excess exercise can have exactly the opposite effect. One of the reasons athletes and sportspeople are so often ill is that the stress and waste products produced by exercise that is too intense can upset the immune system and suppress it. It is important to note that if you are an endurance athlete, or exercising particularly hard or frequently, it is absolutely essential to focus on food quality and to take quality food supplements.

The lymph circulation system has a series of nodes that are like little pockets where lymph fluid is collected and filtered. The immune system works hard in these nodes to clear away any foreign bodies that are dangerous.

It's much more fun to **Live** *it than* **Die***t.*

If these nodes get overloaded with waste they can become inflamed and painful. Your tonsils are a type of lymph node; having inflamed tonsils (tonsillitis) is a symptom of a stressed and overworked lymph system. It used to be common to cut out inflamed tonsils (an operation that would be the equivalent of removing a water treatment plant from the water network because it got clogged up. A pretty silly idea). Much better to reduce the amount of waste in the system.

The lymph system is stimulated by breathing and by movement. Moderate exercise and deep breathing increase its flow and efficiency. It is also stimulated by changes in surface temperature and increases in blood circulation.

Overall, our immune system consists of incredibly effective cells that are perfectly capable of defending us against all manner of 'nasties'. Bacteria, viruses, yeasts, fungi, parasites and cancer are all handled on a daily basis.

The only opponent of our immune systems that we really have to worry about is ourselves. If we overload our system with waste, allow excess toxic debris to collect in a sluggish lymph system, and fail to consume truly nourishing foods containing the vitamins and minerals we need to supply our immune cells, then we fall 'victim' to what we usually term 'infection'. It is then common to try and treat the infection with antibiotics or antivirals. These usually only make the situation worse. They tend to be very general and kill off good bacteria as well as bad. They can cause complete catastrophes in the digestive system by killing off both the good and bad bacteria, leaving a fertile ground for the breeding of yeasts that can penetrate the intestinal wall, allowing through more waste products, and potentially setting up allergic responses.

This vicious cycle of 'infection' from antibiotics to sensitization, to excess waste to more infections to more antibiotics, is a common negative spiral.

A useful reference solution to this conundrum is on the next page.

Give yourself the gift of a strong and powerful immune system

Objective:
To have the strongest, most powerful immune system possible and so ensure that any adverse foreign bodies or wayward cells are dealt with quickly and efficiently.

Benefits:
Freedom from colds and flu, extra energy (not wasted dealing with 'infections'), fewer allergies, lower weight due to less food sensitivity, massive (if not entire) reduction in risk of cancers and inflammatory joint problems.

Strategies:
1. Consume nourishing fruits and vegetables that contain essential immune vitamins – particularly Vitamin C and Beta Carotene (for Vitamin A), as well as immune boosting living plant nutrients.

2. Eat whole grains and whole foods, complete foods that deliver essential immune boosting minerals.

3. Focus on breathing effectively and take moderate exercise to ensure effective lymphatic drainage and power in the lymph system. Do not over-exert yourself, this suppresses the immune system.

4. Take a high quality vitamin and mineral multi-supplement to complement food intake.

5. Drink plenty of clean water to maintain movement of fluids and waste around cells and encourage lymph drainage

6. Make a conscious effort to relax and take time during each day to focus on positive thoughts. Deliberately find things to laugh at. Fart in the bath! (If you still can since you sorted out your digestion!)

7. Eat fresh raw nuts and seeds for essential fats and minerals that are critical to the creation and effective functioning of your immune cells.

8. Avoid nutrient-bereft refined foods, including sugar and refined grains.

9. Avoid contaminated food, including those containing food additives, colours, flavourings, artificial sweeteners and pesticide residues, which all contribute to excess waste in the lymphatic system.

10. Only take medications as an absolute last resort. Avoid antibiotics if at all possible. Take beneficial bowel flora supplements if you have taken antibiotics in the past.

11. Minimize consumption of animal products – they tend to be contaminated with antibiotics and pesticides that can interfere with your bowel function and compromise your immunity.

IT'S ALL INTERCONNECTED –
THE HOLISTIC APPROACH

Your digestion affects the way you feel and think. The way you think and feel affects your digestion.

The cleanliness and efficiency of your liver affects your hormones. Your hormones affect the way your liver behaves.

The amount of energy in your cells affects your appetite for exercise. The amount you exercise affects the energy in your cells.

The strength of your immune system affects how you deal with waste. The amount of waste in your body affects your immune system.

Your digestion affects your immune system. The effectiveness of your immune system affects your digestion.

The amount of energy in your cells affects your cravings for junk and drugs. Your consumption of junk and drugs affects the amount of energy in your cells.

The efficiency of your liver affects your skin. The effectiveness of your skin as a channel of elimination affects your liver.

Everything affects everything.

It is balance, harmony and well-being that your body is trying to achieve and always trying to achieve. In this section we have looked at just a few of the relationships. The relationships are endless. You do not need to know about them all. All you have to do is start to follow your instincts rather than your conscious thoughts when it comes to eating. If you are binging you are probably looking for that short-term 'high' such behaviour gives you. But now you know it comes at the price of a more longer term 'low'.

We have touched on a mere fraction of the miracle that is your body in this section. And what we have touched on is incomplete. We haven't even begun on your gall bladder, spleen, kidneys, brain, or endocrine (hormone) system. Suffice it to say that they are all interconnected. The purpose of this section has been to demonstrate that all body systems and functions are interdependent. And they are all dependent on how and what you eat, how you breathe, how you move and how you feel. If you look at the strategies for blood sugar, digestion, detoxification and skin, you see an emergent pattern, some common threads and elements: the quality of your nourishment; the amount of waste taken in; the cleanliness of tissue fluids; the amount of vitamins and minerals.

You don't need to know it all. You were designed with all the knowledge and instinct you need to get it right. The wild animal does not understand its digestive or immune system – it just eats by instinct. The ants select the living nuts and seeds over the sugar and jam because they rely on their natural senses and latent understanding of what is good for them. Animals in the wild stay healthy; they only start to get diseases, heart problems and cancers when we raise them on farms or in zoos. Man's 'intelligence' is sometimes man's stupidity. Ignorruption!

You have all the resources you need to make all the right decisions. You just need to get back in touch with your genuine hunger, stop being deceived by artificial tastes and smells that disguise drugs and junk as food; and stop taking advice from experts. They so often have a motive or have been educated by someone who has a motive.

The only thing between you and utter perfection
is your beliefs.

Because your beliefs drive your decisions.

And your decisions drive your actions.

And your actions drive your destiny.

Every breath, every sip, every bite, every move,
takes you towards your destiny.

What is the destiny you want?

Decide.

Find the way.

Livetetics.

Live it.

Livetetics: the way

Livetetics:
the way

You are already a master of Livetetics. Livetetics is simply reconnecting with the magical being inside you. A being that was created for perfection – a perfect body, a perfect life, perfect relationships, perfect bliss, perfect strength, perfect vitality, perfect well-being.

Your perfection. True perfection. Not an illusion of perfection that is less than your potential.

Not the illusion of perfection suggested by the editor of a glossy magazine whose job it is to provide an environment in which advertisers want to position their products.

Not the illusion of perfection suggested by the manufacturers of drugs and junk, sold to you as food by associating irrelevant attributes through advertising, packaging, public relations and the creation of interesting, comfortable or 'fun' places to go and buy them.

Not the illusion of perfection suggested by nutritional or medical 'experts' who have been trained in a framework developed by the manufacturers of chemical medicine or adulterated food.

True, unimaginable perfection. Your natural potential. Your true destiny.

The way that follows is just a way of reconnecting. It is not a set of rules and it will be up to you how you follow Livetetic principles. For there is no right or wrong way to live, only the best way for you. You know by now that your choices will determine your outcome.

How deep was your last breath? How straight are you sitting? What was the last thing you put in your mouth?

Your decisions. No one else's.

No one can make you do anything. It is, in the end, always your decision. No-one makes you eat chocolate or crisps or meat, or makes you drink beer or milk. You decide whether or not to eat or drink it.

The people who make chocolate want you to eat it. They want you to associate good things with it, with the smell, the flavour, the texture…

'Go on, treat yourself.' 'Indulge yourself.' 'You're worth it.' 'Pleasure, it is pleasure, pure pleasure.' 'Come and get some, it's fine.' 'Your mother wouldn't mind.' 'Of course it's healthy – it's food.' 'No such thing as an unhealthy food.' 'Makes your mouth water, doesn't it?' 'Go on, just take one little bite…'

'Gotcha!'

If you look at chocolate and see pleasure, that will influence your decision. If you look at chocolate and see pain, that will influence your decision. There is conflict. And you are worried that Livetetics will ask you to give up chocolate, or crisps, or coffee, or alcohol, or meat, or milk, or cheese, or any number of things that you 'can't live without'.

Well, rest easy. You don't have to give up anything that you don't want to. Livetetics is about getting back in touch with your real senses. The senses that are not manipulated by the manufacturers or advertisers. It is only about the decisions that are right for you in the right time for you.

You can go as quickly or as slowly as you like.

There are no calories to count.

No points.

No 'sins'.

Just pure, plain, natural, unadulterated common sense and a means to get back in touch with the extraordinary checks and balances that nature gave you to achieve your ultimate perfection. Livetetics focuses on additions. It is much easier to add things than to take things away. By adding nourishment, your body begins the process of normalization, naturally. So there is no need to give things up. You will naturally start to make better decisions as your body begins to notice what is going on.

Improve digestion, it helps your liver; help your liver it improves your energy; improve your energy, you move more; move more, you improve your digestion.

Improve your breathing, improve your energy. By improving your energy, improve your mood. By improving your mood, improve your digestion. By improving your digestion, improve your liver. By improving your liver, improve your skin. By improving your skin, get more confidence. Meet a partner, have great sex, improve your breathing.

Little positive spirals. Simple things. Easy changes. Fabulous results.

When you are better nourished your tastes will change. When you have more energy your hunger will be different. When you are better balanced you will make better decisions.

Livetetics is not about a big bang. It is not short term.

Incremental, sustainable change. Positive spirals. Just start your spirals spinning in the right direction. It is easy, it is obvious.

It is about life, not death.

Remember – live it, don't diet.

BREATHING

Air is your most vital nutrient. We breathe automatically. If our bodies need to work harder we automatically breathe more deeply. We don't have to think about it.

But, for the most part, we do not breathe efficiently any more. We are shallow breathers and only use a small portion of lung capacity, even when we are exercising.

If you are someone who does participate in an active sport or exercise, try extending the length of your inhalation by 2–3 times while relaxing your muscles into the exercise and notice the immediate drop in your heart rate. It will give you additional energy and reduce the effort you need to expend to keep up the same level of movement.

Using the fullest extent of your lungs is one of the most important steps you can take towards optimal health. It is more important than what you drink and what you eat. Optimizing the amount of oxygen you get into your blood and to your cells influences your metabolism and energy production capacity.

It is easy to improve your lung capacity and improve your breathing. It begins with a very straightforward exercise. You can do this as you read.

Inhale deeply. Hold. Gently, inhale some more. Hold. Gently, inhale some more. Keep going until you cannot comfortably take any more air in and then exhale gently. Keep your shoulders relaxed.

Notice the feeling at the bottom of your lungs where you have used portions of your lungs that you do not normally use.

Do it again.

Sit up. Inhale deeply. Hold. Gently, inhale some more. Hold. Gently, inhale some more. Keep going until you cannot comfortably take any more air in and then exhale gently. Keep your shoulders relaxed.

Now take ten deep breaths, holding each one for a few seconds and then breathing out slowly.

Count as you inhale:

Inhale   1...2...3...4...5
Hold   1...2...3...4...5...6...7...8...9...10
Exhale   1...2...3...4...5...6...7...8...9...10

Do this and notice how you feel. If you overdo it you can feel a little dizzy and light-headed. Do it comfortably. Reduce the number of counts if you like. Or expand them if you like.

A great way to do this is while you are walking. Use your steps for the counts. Inhale over five steps, hold for ten steps, and exhale for ten steps.

In fact, go and do this now. Go and walk – preferably outside – and take ten vital breaths, counting your steps as you do it. Think of something positive with each breath.

The Vital Breathing Technique		
Inhale	Hold	Exhale
1	**2**	**2**
e.g. 5 count/steps	e.g. 10 counts/steps	e.g. 10 counts/steps

Or whatever is comfortable in the same ratio. Build this up with gentle challenges to yourself.

This is the first step of Livetetics. Do this deliberately at least five times a day. Start to experiment with the ratios. Do it as you walk. Inhale for as many steps as is comfortable, hold for as many as is comfortable and then exhale as slowly as is comfortable. Gently challenge yourself to inhale and hold and exhale as long as you comfortably can. Experiment holding for longer, then exhaling fairly quickly. Also try inhaling for as many steps as possible, holding for a short time and then exhaling for as many steps as possible.

But the minimum is ten vital breaths in the 1:2:2 ratio. If five counts is too low then change the count to whatever is comfortable for you to maintain the 1:2:2 ratio for your first ten breaths.

This is very easy to do. It is also very easy not to do!

Do this first thing in the morning and last thing before you rest at night, as well as before your meals: at least five times a day.

WATER

Your body contains about 70 per cent water. You can only last 2–3 days without it. Your cells contain water. The fluids that bathe your cells contain water. Your blood contains water.

Water is an amazing substance. It is a solvent; things dissolve in it. It enables substances to move around your body quickly and efficiently.

Taking in enough clean, fresh water is essential to good health. It enhances the function of a thousand body systems, keeps your cells in good shape and is essential for the condition of your skin.

Yet most of us are completely out of touch with our thirst. If you get as far as feeling thirsty you are likely to be seriously dehydrated. Most people do not deliberately drink water and many never consume any water at all. A survey of 37,000 people in the UK, undertaken by my nutrition consultancy a couple of years ago, showed that one in ten people don't make any deliberate effort at all to drink water. More than half drink less than half of what they need and only 15 per cent have enough.

Yet drinking water is probably one of the most powerful changes that can be made to your intake. It increases energy, improves skin condition, helps you wake up refreshed, improves concentration and memory, and makes it easier to lose weight.

Not drinking enough can lead to increased headaches and migraine, bad breath, bad hair (greasy, dull or dry), poor vision, joint pain, backache, sweet cravings, indigestion, constipation, mood swings, depression, anxiety, high blood pressure and impotence.

Any government minister with any health remit reading this should insist immediately on clinical trials on all drugs and medications used for headaches, migraine, joint pain, indigestion, backache, impotence, depression, anxiety and constipation. The trial should compare the efficacy of the drugs versus a placebo, with the placebo group split between a group that is encouraged to drink seven to eight glasses of pure, fresh water every day and a group that is not.

The results would be extraordinary. My experience suggests that pure water is more effective in these and a myriad of other conditions than prescribed medications. Next to air, it is your most important nutrient.

Why have clinical trials for conditions using water never taken place? Why are they never likely to take place? Because there isn't any money in prescribing water! Pharmaceutical manufacturers can only make money if they can provide evidence of the efficacy and safety of their medications. To protect their medications from being copied they need to patent the formulations. You can't patent things that are already in the public domain. Nobody can patent water! So no research is done, no comparisons are made, and people continue to take medications for conditions they could cure with water.

Ignorruption. Look at and publicise a collection of evidence (research) that is too narrow and you can get intelligent people to do some really dumb things.

But don't take my word for it. Try it for yourself. There is no point having your body in a sticky, polluted mess. Water is the universal solvent. Virtually everything that moves in your body is dissolved in water.

Good hydration is essential to your well-being. It helps keep lymph clear and moving, and enables the carriage of fat residues and toxic debris away from cells and out of the body.

Drink a minimum of seven glasses a day of pure fresh, unadulterated water. Drink a variety: filtered, distilled or good quality bottled mineral water. Use a wide variety if possible. If the only thing available is tap water then, subject to your being in a country where it is 'safe', it is better to drink it than not!

Minimum 7 glasses of water a day	
	Increase amount drunk gently and comfortably
• 1 on rising	Use small glasses at the beginning
• 1 before breakfast	Always drink water before any food or snack ideally 10–20 mins before
• 1 mid morning	
• 1 before lunch	Fine to add a little fresh squeezed juice – try fresh lemon in the morning
• 1 mid afternoon	Use cranberry juice or powder 2–3 times a day if you're going for fat reduction
• 1 before dinner	
• 1 on retiring	Herbal teas are a good idea – avoid teas with colourings or flavourings both 'natural' and 'artificial'.
	Avoid drinking while you eat.

Adulterated water doesn't count! As you see above, your water tally does not include sodas, squash, milk or milk shakes, stimulant drinks, tea, coffee, alcohol or concentrated fruit juices.

While I was writing this book, one of the world's largest manufacturers of cola and sugared soft drinks was in the news. This company had launched a new 'designer' water onto the UK market. It turned out that the water came from the local water board tap in Swindon and there was uproar about this; that a company would charge about 1,000 times the price for water, even if it had been through some advanced filtering process and been packaged in some snazzy bottles.

Why the uproar? Why would it be any different to sell tap water that had been filtered, from selling tap water that has been contaminated with sugar, colourings, flavourings and preservatives? It's tap water just the same!

It's exactly what we've come to accept as 'normal' or 'OK'. We have been led to believe, after years of advertising, that a brown, fizzy liquid contaminated with ten teaspoons of sugar is 'refreshing', 'a treat', 'relaxing', or whatever nonsense the brand custodians could think would motivate us to buy it.

But now the contaminated water producers (soft drink manufacturers) have realized that consumers are on to them. People are becoming aware that the polluted solutions in the brightly coloured cans, sold in icy cold glasses, are not actually as good as the imagery suggests. Enlightened consumers are learning that these chemical-ridden concoctions rob them of energy, make them fat and potentially give them life-threatening diseases. So, to exploit this new consumer awareness, the junk manufacturers are trying to sell us things that are actually beneficial, like plain water, and then they get criticized for it!

As a fellow marketing man I have great sympathy for the junk salesmen. They have a tough road ahead. After 100 years of incrementally cajoling people into eating more and more contaminated food (refined 'food' polluted with sugar, salt, fat, flavourings, colourings, etc) they are gradually having to accept that they are left with consumers who are addicted to rubbish that makes them sick.

And so the marketing men have to try and manage their way out of the situation by gradually creating brands and products that appeal to consumers' needs for real vitality and well-being, rather than the shallow illusion they have peddled for so long. But these consumers have acquired tastes (or even addictions) for the contaminated foods: salt, sugar, fat, flavourings. Consumers have been educated into wanting 'taste' and 'texture' and 'convenience'.

When it comes to quenching thirst there is nothing like plain, fresh water, drunk slowly at body temperature, enjoying every sip. It's hard to create a brand with enough differentiation to make money. But you can expect a lot to try over the coming years. Watch out for 'designer' water, 'smart' water, 'enhanced' water, 'sexy' water, 'weird, colourful-label' water. And, of course, a lot of it will be sold in plastic containers that may leach chemicals into the water, and which in turn will have to be disposed of;

hopefully in an environmentally friendly way.

As for you, drink that variety. Filter your own. Get bottled water if you can trust the sources. Collect your own rainwater and filter it. But, whatever you do…

Drink seven glasses of water a day.

Easy to do. Easy not to do.

Keep doing what you've always done and you'll keep getting what you've always got. If you do this and a lot of your 'disease' conditions go away then write to me and let me know. Between us we may protect our children and grandchildren from unnecessary medications.

FRUIT

Fruit is perfect food. Fresh, organic, ripe fruit is about as pure a food as you can eat and is a fantastic source of nourishment for every body system. It supplies vitamins, minerals, living water and important plant nutrients that are absolutely essential in a lean healthy body. We are only just beginning to learn how essential these living plant nutrients are.

Your target is five pieces a day but more is fine if you want it. As an absolute minimum, you should eat three portions of fruit a day.

The grid below shows which fruits are best. Some release sugar slower than others and these are best to help you lose fat and avoid laying it down. Variety is critical. Try to make every piece of fruit different. If you eat more than five pieces a day select the extra pieces only from the A list.

Category A – As much as you like			
Cherries	Apple	Peach	Fresh pineapple juice
Grapefruit	Plum	Orange	Fresh grapefruit juice
Pear	Fresh apple juice	Grapes	
Category B – In moderation			
Fresh orange juice	Fruit cocktail	Apricots	Cantaloupe melon
Kiwifruit	Mango	Pawpaw	
Banana	Sultanas	Pineapple	
Category C – Keep to a minimum			
Watermelon	Dried fruit		

Preferably eat fruit before a meal, to allow it to digest cleanly and to prepare your digestive system. Fruit is digested quickly and cleanly. If it gets stuck in the digestive system with other food it can literally go rotten and ferment in your gut.

Many people who say they 'don't like fruit' have experienced negative effects from eating fruit in the wrong way. There are always one or two fruits that you will find you like. One way to find out which ones appeal to you most is to go on a long, remote walk. Take nothing to eat or drink except a bag of various fresh fruits. Walk for as long as it takes to get your hunger to Level One (you are hungry and cannot feel any presence of food in your system from a previous meal.) Remember to use the opportunity to play around with your breathing, counting with your steps and noticing the breathing rhythm that works best for you. Sit on the top of your hill, or in the middle of the woods and, thirsty and hungry, select a piece of fruit.

Take a small bite and savour it. Chew it at least fifty times and notice how it disappears from your mouth without you needing to consciously swallow it. Revel in the natural juices and notice how refreshing they are. Try fruits you don't normally buy or like and notice how they feel when you eat them.

Then, just before you have had enough, lie down, shut your eyes and feel your digestive system process the fruit. Feel the fire burn and notice how this living energy is transferred to your body from the fruit. You are experiencing a truly 'functional' food.

'Functional' food; you have no doubt come across the phrase. It is being bandied about the food industry as a new paradigm in food manufacture. To add things to food that have specific 'functions'. The most commonly seen so far include the processed margarines that contain chemicals that are designed to lower blood pressure, and the sweet dairy products that contain 'friendly bacteria'. One that always amuses me, as well, is the category of high sugar sodas to which caffeine has been added to give you a lift; these deadly concoctions are peddled and thought to be in the 'well-being' category.

The only really functional foods are those that nature created, to which nothing has been added and from which nothing has been taken away.

Refined and processed foods are invariably dysfunctional because they have had nutrients removed and have contaminants added. The term 'functional food' would be better termed 'less dysfunctional food'. It is evidence that the food manufacturers are trying to give us a bit of well-being by making their depleted and contaminated concoctions slightly less damaging.

Beware of processed fruit juices. They are rarely 'fresh'. Many processed juices are made from concentrate and they are pasteurized. That is they are treated by intense heat to stop the juice going 'off' so quickly. This dramatically reduces the beneficial 'living energy' of the juice. Most carton juices contain pasteurized juices. These juices are often fast sugar releasers and provide a fraction of the potential nutrition of the real fruit.

They are however useful. They can add flavour to water and, especially at the beginning, people often find that water is hard to drink because they think it doesn't have any flavour. If your palate is conditioned to the intense taste of ten spoons of sugar in a glass of water (like a cola) then pure water takes a while to taste as good as it is. Processed juices can be useful. They also provide some of the beneficial nutrients from the fruit but it is best to dilute them; 25 per cent juice to water is ideal.

Best, however, is to take fresh, raw juices in preference to processed, heat-treated juice or juice made from a concentrate.

But back to our fruit. Five pieces a day. Don't get hung up about what a 'portion' is. It's approximately one apple or a handful of grapes. See what works for you.

Organic fruit is best if you can get it. But don't avoid fruit if you can't find quality organics. It is better to eat chemically fertilized fruit with pesticide residues than not to eat it at all. Just make sure you wash it well. Fruit brings living nutrients that aid in detoxification, and essential nutrients for energy, fat metabolism and immunity.

Most tinned fruits come contaminated with sugar syrups and they have been heat-treated. Conventional guidelines suggest that these count as a portion of fruit but they do not meet Livetetic standards. Processed and cooked fruits do not offer the same benefits as fresh, raw fruit. Your five portions should all be fresh and raw.

Sounds a lot? Here's what a day might look like:

What and when	Portions
Squeeze two fresh lemons and have them in a glass of water on rising. In winter you might like to prepare this with hot water and add a spoon of organic honey	1
Grate an apple into your breakfast cereal or porridge. Or eat a pear before breakfast	1
Have a handful of grapes with your mid-morning water	1
Eat an orange with your mid-afternoon water	1
Have a banana and soy smoothie with ground nuts before daily exercise/movement	1

If you want to lose weight, it is a good idea to consider fruit smoothies made with fruit, soy yoghurt or soy milk, adding a couple of cubes of tofu and a sprinkling of finely ground nuts and seeds. This adds a little protein that can slow the sugar release without unduly compromising the speed of digestion. Soy products tend to be much lower in fat and contaminants than dairy products and the soy-based proteins are easier on the digestion, as well as providing additional beneficial nutrients. Dairy proteins slow down digestion more markedly and so can compromise the beneficial effects of the fruit. It is best never to mix the consumption of fruit or fruit juice with any animal products (meat, fish, eggs or dairy).

Remember there are calories and there are calories. There is fake 'energy' and there is real energy. Fresh fruit provides real energy. It stokes your furnace and lifts your metabolism. It helps you process fat and it sets up a positive spiral. Because it is rich in living waters it provides all the benefits you get from water with extra benefits to skin, hair and nails, even more relief from depression and anxiety, and profound improvements on digestion. People who eat enough fruit have much better skin and rarely get stretch marks.

Three portions of fruit contain about the same number of calories as a chocolate-based snack bar. There is no comparison, though, on the nutritional profile. The fruit contains living water, lots of vitamins, essential fibre and important plant nutrients. The chocolate snack contains excesses of fat, salt and no fibre or living fluids.

If you are accustomed to a cup of tea and/or a little treat during the day, don't try to stop with willpower and self-denial; just have a glass of water and a piece of fruit first. For most, the need for the junk disappears as the body becomes nourished and re-balanced. Even if you still fancy a bit of your regular junk, then at least after the juice and water you stand a chance of dealing with its empty calories.

Five pieces of fruit a day. More if you like.

Easy to do. Easy not to do.

Make a picture of your destiny. Feel how it will feel when you have achieved your perfection. What will you say to yourself when you stand in front of the mirror and you have achieved your perfect proportions, YOUR perfect proportions. How great will it feel? And you will have achieved it simply by living at your optimal health and well-being.

Remember every breath, every sip, every bite, every move takes a decision. Your decision. You decide your destiny, no one else.

Add the breathing, add the water, add the fruit. Adding things is easy. Once you achieve nourishment, balance and well-being then the best decisions will come easily.

It is utterly pointless to go on a 'calorie-controlled diet' without adjusting the type of calories you eat. The cravings for junk come because you are malnourished and out of balance. To get rid of the cravings you need to be nourished and balanced, then perfection will come as if by magic.

Livetetics.

No counting.

No willpower.

No diets.

Go and get a piece of fruit. Enjoy it.

VEGETABLES

C hildren, in their natural state, will make sensible food choices. They will eat fruit and salad and vegetables readily, with great enjoyment. Unfortunately, and in the western world particularly, by the time children can hold a knife and fork, their palates have virtually been destroyed by empty calorie junk, chemical flavours, excess fat, and far too much salt and sugar with everything.

Like fruit, vegetables are virtually perfect food. They are packed with essential vitamins, minerals, fibre and vital plant nutrients. They also contain essential protein including all of the essential amino acids.

Vegetables are best eaten raw, gently boiled or steamed (without salt!) or stir-fried with a little organic virgin olive oil. They make fantastic soups, casseroles and hot pots. Try dressing vegetables with oil and vinegar dressings or make interesting sauces for added interest, flavour and nutrition. Try adapting your old favourite pasta sauces and trying them on vegetables. Fantastic! Green beans, courgettes and shredded spring greens with any pasta sauce make a meal far more nutritious than the equivalent made with refined flour pasta.

Children must eat vegetables. So must you. This isn't a 'should' or an 'ought', it is a 'must'.

'I know I should eat my vegetables', goes the protest, 'but I've never liked them and I just can't get around to liking them.' This is largely a conditioned response and it often goes back to childhood. Hours spent staring at heads of broccoli on a plate with the threat that if they weren't eaten there would be no ice-cream! This was not a good way to set up positive associations with vegetables and salad; to establish them as barriers to enjoyment, hurdles to be jumped to get at what you really liked.

Your mother would get angry with you if you didn't eat them. She wanted to reward you with the junk dessert but she knew you ought to eat the vegetables. Maybe you weren't hungry – that would be fine – but then you didn't need to be hungry for ice cream, it would just glide down, pure good flavour and sugar and fat and lacking in any substance. It was pure pleasure with no requirement for being 'hungry'.

And so we set up negative associations with the green stuff. It is 'cool' to eat crisps, and sweets and chocolate but it is 'soft' to eat vegetables. 'Hard' cops on television flout the laws of nutrition and demonstrate how 'tough' they are by eating junk and laughing at the 'hippy faddists' who care about what they put in their bodies.

Vegetables do not have any brand presence. There is no advertising for vegetables every morning on the television, persuading children that these are the foundations for brains, muscles, bones, energy, strength, agility, stamina, endurance and ability.

It is sugary cereals, milk chocolate buttons, coloured gelatine sweeties, processed fish fingers, more sugary cereals, white chocolate bars, high salt and saturated fat potato crisps. It goes on and on, and on and on, and on. Millions of pounds worth of incessant propaganda, pictures of fun and adventure, sports celebrities, pop stars, glamour, fashion and desire.

Remember this one? Sing along with me…

'A finger of junk is just enough
To give your kids a treat
A finger of junk is just enough until it's time to eat
It's full of [imaginary] goodness
And very small and neat
A finger of junk is just enough
To give your kids a treat.'

Or we were given pictures of the countryside, of farmers and harvesting, of sunshine and crops; incessant pictures of goodness tag-lined with:

'A junk bar a day helps you work rest and play.'

And it's not just children who are targeted...

'It's the honeycomb middle that weighs so little!'

... went the slim girl in the swimsuit as she got out of the pool, patted her flat tummy and smiled to the camera.

But how are the children, the people, to decide? The constant barrage of junk advertising is conditioning our children. Conditioning them to accept that these products are fine as part of a 'healthy balanced (or varied) diet'. And the products appear on the government 'food group' charts as part of the 'carbohydrate group' or the 'dairy group'. The packets contain no useful information about how much is safe. Any attempt to restrict advertising or encourage useful labels is met by the cries of the food lobbies...

'Oh no', they say,' we are good guys'. 'We only sell things that people like. The advertising doesn't make people want to buy more. We only do it so they buy our brand. It doesn't expand the market for junk.'

Meanwhile the account executives in the advertising agencies are telling their junk 'food' clients to advertise, advertise, advertise. 'Noise' (lots of advertising) in a category will keep the market buoyant and growing.

The junk manufacturers wheel out research that is aggregated to show that our children are eating the same number of calories that they ever have. When the government gets worried about the levels of obesity, early onset of diabetes, early incidence of heart disease and autistic spectrum disorders (from Attention Deficit Hyperactive Disorder and dyslexia to more significant mental problems), the junk makers' response is 'It isn't to do with how much children are eating – look at this chart – they are eating the same as before. It's just that they don't exercise, that's the problem!'

The ministers are too busy to look at the figures in detail to see how much more sugar, salt, fat, chemical sweeteners, flavourings and colourings are going down the necks of our children. The legislators back away. The food lobbies are very powerful, better not mess with them. Leave things as they are…

And the ignorruption goes on. The children eat the junk. It tastes good. It is designed to taste good. It appeals to their evolutionary instincts for salt and fat and sugar and it contains chemical flavourings that have been researched to tickle little taste buds. And they eat it. And it contains no nourishment – not true nourishment – and they can't tell when they've had enough because there is no substance to the junk and their stomachs don't signal to them to stop in time. And when they sit down to a meal they won't eat their vegetables, not unless they are disguised in some way that is colourful, salty, fatty and sweet. How many parents have come through my door who give their kids buttered vegetables with ketchup, as 'It's the only way I can get them down'. Are we surprised?

There is no choice in this matter. Five portions of vegetables are required every day. It is a must, not a should. It is essential. Green leafy and highly coloured vegetables are to be the most prized. They provide essential components that aid detoxification, critical minerals, vitamins, fibre, protein and living plant nutrients.

You can eat as much as you like. Just focus on variety and, if you're eating more than five, then stay in group A. These release sugar more slowly and are the most fat-loss friendly.

Take care not to overcook your vegetables, treat them gently. If you boil or steam, consider using the water as a stock for soups to capture any nutrients that have leached out. As always, organic and in season is best, but variety is the key. Experiment with new varieties, grow your own. Vegetables and salads provide the ultimate living food for living health.

Category A – As much as you like			
Artichoke hearts	Chicory	Mange tout	Spring onions
Asparagus spears	Chillies	Marrow	Tomatoes
Aubergine	Chinese leaves	Mushrooms	Turnip
Bamboo shoots	Courgettes	Mustard and cress	Water chestnuts
Bean sprouts	Cucumber	Okra	Watercress
Broccoli	Fennel	Onions	Peas
Brussels sprouts	French (Dwarf) beans	Pepper, red, green	
Cabbage	Garlic	or yellow	
Cauliflower	Kale	Radishes	
Celeriac	Leeks	Runner beans	
Celery	Lettuce	Spinach	
Category B – In moderation			
Carrots	Potato, new	Beets	Potato, boiled
Yam	Sweetcorn	Swede	Sweet potato
Category C – Keep to a minimum			
Pumpkin	Potato, baked	Parsnips	French fries

As ever, tinned and processed vegetables are second best by a long way. They are overheated and invariably contaminated with sugar and salt. Many tins have unstable plastic coatings that leach potentially hormone-disrupting chemicals into the contents.

As for the children, give them salad and vegetables ahead of the meal, just after their piece of fruit. If and when they eat their vegetables then give them the rest of the meal you were planning. If they don't eat it then assume they are not hungry and let them go about their business.

But don't, under any circumstances, allow the junk snacks in between meals. Definitely not if the fruit and vegetables are not going down. Don't worry, no child will ever starve themselves if there is food around. However, if there is junk around, it will invariably be selected instead of the food and then semi-starvation can take place.

Use exactly the same strategy yourself. Breathe, then water, then fruit, then vegetables. Only eat more if you are still really hungry.

Fruit and vegetables are real food. They are about nourishment, life, strength, energy, intelligence, flexibility, being good at games, strong bones and teeth (green leafy vegetables are a better source of calcium than dairy products; they come with synergistic minerals and vitamins and do not contain excess protein and fat).

Fruit and vegetables are food. Junk is junk. Junk without food is death, food without junk is life, and food with junk is somewhere in between. Most children can understand this, they don't want to be manipulated any more than you do. You can understand it too.

The main issue here is to re-establish your palate. Vegetables are absolutely delicious. They have some of the most subtle and intricate flavours you can imagine. But it takes a bit of time to get your palate back after the chemical onslaught that most of us have had to endure.

Many children, after bottle feeding and eating from processed food jars, have no natural palate at all. This can make it almost impossible to feed them any fresh or raw food. Compound it with confectionery, crisps, processed fish fingers, nuggets, pizza slices and oven chips and you send them down the slippery chute to diabetes, heart disease and cancer.

Soups, casseroles, hot pots, stir fries, kebabs, salads, chopped vegetables with interesting dips; there are many ways to do it and hundreds of cookery books that can inspire you on your new path.

It must be done. Find a way.

Do it and succeed. Fail to do it and fail.

Your life.

Your decisions.

Decide.

(And don't expect much help from the government within 25 years. The junk labels may be starting to get health warnings, but only in the simplest of terms. It will take many years before this message is believed and broadcast as it should be.)

WHOLE GRAINS

Whole grains are powerhouses of nutrition. They haven't been around that long in our diets from an evolutionary point of view – just 5,000 to 10,000 years – a mere blink compared with the length of time we have been evolving. But whole grains can be a good source of a large range of nutrients.

Whole grains contain complete carbohydrates that release their sugars more slowly and evenly than their 'refined' cousins and have the added advantage of bringing with them the vitamins and minerals needed to process them. They are fabulous sources of protein in the right amounts so that the digestion process is efficient and has minimal toxic by-products. This is good for the liver and kidneys and lets them get on with the more important aspects of cleaning the system, rather than dealing with unwanted residues from excess protein in meals.

There are loads of grains, many of which you may never have enjoyed. They are a cornerstone of the Livetetic way.

Whole grains provide fabulous sources of vitamins, minerals and protein. There are so many varieties and recipes for them that you can never get bored. Start to experiment with whole grains and let your imagination and creativity run riot.

You are aiming at 2–5 servings of whole grains a day. The amount will be determined by your hunger, not by me! Use your hunger scale to get a feel for what works for you. Because whole grains contain nourishment and fibre they trigger your body's normal hunger mechanisms and it is virtually impossible to overeat them.

Some obese people are now going for surgery to reduce the size of their stomachs or have plastic bags of water or oil surgically implanted in their stomachs so they are physically unable to eat enough food to make

...cornerstones of Livetetics

them fat. This is self-induced starvation. A far simpler way to get exactly the same result is to eat whole foods that have more substance and bulk than the refined junk in processed foods. Whole foods work with your body – refined foods work against you. If you eat fresh, healthy whole grains you can eat until you are satisfied, never go hungry and your body will naturally balance itself over time.

I find that clients are amazed by this when they start eating whole grains. First of all they don't realize how many types there are, and secondly they are amazed at how satisfying they are. They have a texture that lends itself to chewing – satisfying in itself – and a wide range of rich, nutty flavours that really spring out at you once your natural palate is restored.

As for children, grains are fantastic. They are easy to eat, and can be used to form the basis of burgers or nuggets, as well as being a great way of serving vegetables. Vegetables chopped into a bed of whole grains with a rich, tasty sauce, using tomatoes and interesting herbs and spices, is a winner with children and adults.

A variety of whole grains will deliver all the protein you need as part of a Livetetic menu and will do so in the absence of excess fat. Whole grains are great for your heart and blood and provide a fantastic source of long-lasting energy.

Category A – If you want a little more			
Quinoa	Brown rice		
Category B – In moderation			
Wheat	Rice, white	Cornmeal	Oats
Buckwheat	Pasta, wholemeal	Couscous	Bulgar
Barley	Rye		
Category C – Keep to a minimum			
Millet	Tapioca	Rice/corn pasta	

WHOLE GRAINS • 207

A note of caution with whole grains: Western diets include a lot of wheat. Wheat is a staple but a lot of people demonstrate intolerance to the gluten found in it and other gluten grains (barley, rye, oats, triticale, spelt and kamut).

Avoiding wheat and wheat products can be difficult but for some it can be absolutely essential. Do not worry too much about this, especially at the beginning: there is enough to think about. But it is a good idea to limit wheat to one serving a day and preferably not to eat wheat every day. So try to use wheat at one meal only and not more than four times a week.

BREAD

B reads can be a handy way of getting your grains. But take care, grain breads are often still predominantly wheat, so check ingredients and don't overdo them. Wheat is a potential fat-loss blocker and gluten grains can cause problems for a lot of people. Avoid breads that use refined/white flours.

Category A – If you want a little more			
Barley bread	Oat bran bread	Pumpernickel	
Rye bread	Mixed grain bread		
Category B – In moderation			
Bulgar bread	Brown bun	Barley flour bread	Wheat bread,
Linseed rye bread	Semolina bread	Melba toast	Wholegrain
Pitta bread	Oat bread		
Category C – Keep to a minimum			
Wheat bread	Bread stuffing	French baguette	
Bagel	Gluten-free bread		

We're going for 3–5 servings of whole grains a day. A serving is about half a cup of cooked grain or rice, or one piece of bread or toast. Keep gluten grains to a maximum of one serving a day. The gluten grains are barley, rye, oats, triticale, spelt and kamut.

Easy to do. Grains go with anything and can be used in many recipes. If you have recipes that you love based on meat or fish, just substitute the meat with grains and root vegetables. You'll get a much healthier meal that works with you rather than against you.

Do it!

PULSES/BEANS

Pulses and beans (legumes) are wonderful sources of useful protein and complex, energy-giving carbohydrates. They come with a good supply of essential fatty acids. Sprouting beans, in particular, have a dramatically increased protein content and there are sprouted bean mixes available at good health food stores.

It is best to buy your beans and pulses and soak and cook them yourself. Watch the directions on the packet: certain beans must be hard boiled for at least ten minutes to ensure that they are safe to eat. Canned varieties are a fall-back. If you do go for cans, get them unsalted and rinse off the water thoroughly. However, canned beans really are only second best and home preparation is so easy that they are really not worth the extra cost. The tinned varieties are usually unnecessarily contaminated with sugar and salt.

Pulses make an excellent base and thickener for hearty soups, broths and casseroles. They are incredibly versatile. Enjoy experimenting. Seasoned bean spreads can make excellent sandwich fillers.

Category A – As much as you like			
Soya beans	Lentils	Lima beans	Pinto beans
Kidney beans	Butter beans	Chick peas	Black-eyed beans
Haricot/navy beans			
Category B – In moderation			
Kidney beans, tinned	Lentils, green, tinned		
Category C – Keep to a minimum			
Broad beans	Baked beans, canned		

Alongside grains and vegetables, 3–5 portions of legumes will deliver all of the carbohydrate and protein you need in an easily digestible form.

Legumes are extraordinarily versatile. With grains they will easily replace meat or chicken in virtually any favourite dish and they will deliver more rounded nourishment without all the excess fat and cholesterol delivered by animal products. They add substance and texture to soups, casseroles, pies and hotpots.

Children love legumes and, as a transition, you can 'disguise' them by mashing them into patties or nuggets along with grains and vegetables.

Sadly given a bad press by associations with the 'hippy' crowd, pulses and beans are powerhouses of energy and nourishment that are essential for growth and repair and stoking the all-important digestive furnace. They also aid the liver and kidneys by reducing the toxic burden of diets that are based too heavily on protein from animals.

Beans and pulses, with their complementary proteins and living nutrition, are a vital component of Livetetic nourishing intake. Alongside the grains and vegetables, they provide all the protein you need in a highly digestible format with hardly any fat.

3–5 servings a day.

Easy to do. Easy not to do.

Your destiny.

Your choice.

ESSENTIAL FATS

A word about fat: you don't need much! There is an average requirement for about the equivalent of a dessertspoon daily of essential fat. Roughly the amount you would spread on a piece of toast.

All other fat is excess to requirements. The body can make fat from carbohydrates if it needs to.

Essential fatty acids are essential for lean body health. The best sources are clean, organic seed oils, nuts and seeds or oily fish (if only you could find clean, uncontaminated fish!)

A good oil blend ensures you get benefits from these essential oils. A tablespoon once or twice a day as part of a salad dressing is a great way to use it. Alternatively, blend into smoothies, add to vegetables or stir into sauces just before serving.

Never cook with these oils and keep them refrigerated in airtight containers. They are pure and sensitive oils and need to be taken care of. One amazing side effect of these oils will be the improvement you will notice in skin condition. It would be worth trading any normal external skin treatments while you start to introduce these essential oils into your body and notice the difference.

A note on 'low fat' labelling. We have touched on this before, but be wary of unscrupulous manufacturers who exploit the ignorance of unwary shoppers.

Oil Blends – 1-2 tablespoons a day			
A quality organic oil blend with a combination of cold pressed, unrefined seed oils			
Oils –Or you could prepare your own blend			
Flax oil	Unprocessed	Unprocessed	Unprocessed corn oil
Hemp oil	sunflower oil	safflower oil	Wheatgerm oil

The 'low-fat' food scam

'Low Fat' foods can soon be HIGH FAT on your waist and thighs.

You can hardly walk past a food aisle these days without brightly wrapped 'foods' screaming out at you 'Low Fat', 'Reduced Fat', 'Only 2 per cent Fat', '97 per cent Fat Free'. The packaging suggests to you that it might be all right to eat these even if you're trying to rid yourself of the odd fatty bulge.

Do NOT be taken in.

Companies that make these claims may be telling the 'truth' but they are peddling an image: the wrong image. They intend to exploit the ignorance of the average consumer who believes that 'low fat' versions of foods are OK to eat when they are making healthy diet choices. Regrettably, this is not usually true.

Why? You ask.

Well, one thing that food manufacturers want you to do is eat the products they make. They are not responsible for what those foods do to you. The unscrupulous ones will do anything they can to get their products into your shopping basket. Current statistics suggest that around 58 per cent of the UK population are overweight or obese and marketing research shows that we are becoming more and more concerned about the quality of the foods we eat. At any one time it is estimated that 50 per cent of women are actively on a diet, and it's been reported that around 95 per cent of those diets fail.

So if you are the manufacturer of a food that is likely to pile on the pounds and make people fat, what are you to do? You have to make a claim on the packaging that would encourage shoppers to continue putting your products in their mouths.

Enter the 'low fat' scam: this confidence trick involves making a claim about the quantity of fat in a product and using that to imply that it might be a healthy product or may assist you to lose weight. In most cases this is not true.

Food manufacturers know that people must like the products they make. There are three evolutionary cravings that they often use to peddle their products: our natural cravings for fat, salt and sugar. In the natural world, foods containing sugars, fats and salt are highly prized and usually highly nutritious. In the manufactured food world, these components are added in bulk without the associated nutrition. As we know, they provide 'empty' calories but they help sell junk food!

To make a 'low fat' or 'reduced' claim, all the manufacturers have to do is reformulate the product with less fat or state how much fat is in the packet. They do not have to tell you that in most cases they have replaced the missing fat with extra sugars and, usually, added chemical flavourings to try and trick your tongue into liking its taste.

All excess sugar turns to fat!

Low fat foods are often very high in empty sugars. Wherever you see 'Low Fat' you should understand that it may be low fat in the packet but it is likely very soon to be HIGH FAT in your body.

Another trick is to adjust the weight of a high fat food by adding other ingredients that do not contain fat. How can this be done?

Well, imagine you were selling butter, 100 per cent fat. If you were to blend a knob of butter into a glass of water so that 90 per cent of the weight was water, then you could say that only ten per cent of the weight was fat, even though 100 per cent of the calories were derived from fat. And so the water and butter solution could proclaim '90 per cent fat free'.

Yet another trick along these lines is to inject meat and chicken products with water and textured proteins. This makes them heavier (they can be sold for more) and allows for misleading low fat claims

Best advice is usually to avoid any food carrying a 'low fat' claim. Invariably, they are misleading you. The legislators are catching on but, as ever, ignorruption is rife and the lobbies are most effective at confusing the politicians. It only takes a few experts, an 'independent' nutrition organization and some massaging of the aggregated statistics, and you can throw the government off the scent for years.

Damaged/mutated fats

Processed foods are often contaminated with mutated fats: vegetable oils that have been heated. Hydrogenated fats (chemically produced soft fats) and other manufactured and processed fats have chemical structures that can have damaging effects. Watch out for these junk fats in processed food and bakery products. They have no place in a healthy body. Fortunately you will avoid these junk fats if you avoid the empty calories junk sold as food in the bakery section of any 'food' store.

NUTS AND SEEDS

Nuts and seeds are among nature's superfoods. They are packed with essential minerals and essential fats. Use them for snacking or grind them onto cereal, salads or into smoothies. Eat them raw and fresh. Peanuts don't count and don't eat roasted or salted nuts or seeds. Roasted, salted nuts are full of damaged fats and are loaded with salt.

Have a handful a day of mixed nuts and seeds. Keep them refrigerated in airtight containers.

Nuts and nut butters – A handful/couple of tablespoons			
Brazil nuts	Walnuts	Pistachio nuts	Cashew nuts
Hazel nuts	Pecan nuts		
Seeds –In the same handful			
Sunflower	Pumpkin	Sesame	

They can be added to soups and casseroles, ground into meal for bread or pancakes, mixed in with cake batters or when you make biscuits. Fabulous!

In small quantities, fresh, raw nuts and seeds are nature's powerhouses. Carry some with you all the time.

EXTRA PROTEIN

M any of my clients express concern about 'getting enough protein' from vegetables, grains and legumes. They don't want to become 'vegetarians'.

There is a great deal of nonsense flung around about protein. I find often that people have been misled to believe that vegetable sources of protein are 'inferior' or lower 'quality' than animal sources. The body is perfectly capable of getting all of the protein it requires from these plant-based food sources.

The 'official' protein 'food group' is dominated by pictures of meat and fish and eggs. All are superfluous to protein requirements. All of the essential amino acids are perfectly adequately covered by the plant-based protein sources. They are much more easily digested, come with a wider range of vitamins, minerals and enzymes and contain far less fat.

The notion that animal products are essential components of a healthy intake is a complete fabrication. They can be included, by all means, but they must be in very small quantities. Animal products are hard on the digestion and produce a lot of acidic and toxic by-products that put a strain on the liver and kidneys. They are low in fibre and high in fat. Consistent meat and dairy eaters are more prone to degenerative diseases, carry more weight and have weaker bones. Excess protein delivered by animal products can cause the body to leach essential minerals from the bones to buffer the acid by-products of their digestion.

In addition, animals are at the top of the food chain. And the chain of modern animal husbandry can be a very unhealthy chain indeed. Gone are the days when animals and chickens foraged on fields and roamed freely to get adequate exercise. Now they are confined to small areas, fed chemically 'enhanced' feeds, injected with antibiotics and growth hormones and often even fed the remnants of other dead animals.

Modern meat is potentially a ghastly concoction of dangerous proteins, pesticides, hormone and antibiotic residues and excess fat. It is best avoided altogether or taken in utmost moderation.

Anyone who cares about the wider effects of their food consumption should also spare a thought for those who are starving in our world. The production of animal-derived foods is highly inefficient. It is perhaps only useful if ruminant animals are allowed to roam free over areas of land on which it is quite impossible to grow crops. But grain-feeding cattle takes 8–15 kilos of grain to produce a kilo of meat. It is a ridiculously inefficient way to produce food and it is robbing the poor in this world of their lives. When you sit down to a meat meal you are depriving people of the nourishment they need to survive. If we were to turn the agricultural land currently devoted to raising cattle over to the indigenous peoples of the countries where it is happening, a great deal of hardship would be alleviated. The environmental effects of cattle production, from farm slurry to methane production, also impose serious global pollution problems.

You don't have to label yourself 'vegetarian'; such labels are not helpful. Simply adjust your balance of intake to one that works with your body and is in harmony with the environment rather than against it. Eating a little meat and fish can still be part of what you do if you really feel you 'need' it, but the fruit, vegetable, grain and legume groups will deliver all the protein you need.

There is one potential anomaly: Vitamin B12 is abundant in flesh foods but is no longer found in our vegetable food. In the natural world, the action of bacteria in the soil would make for the adequate consumption of B12 from the roots of vegetables that would be eaten imperfectly clean. Nowadays, if you move to a vegetable- and plant-based intake, B12 will need to come from fortification or a minimal consumption of animal foods.

'What about fish?' you may cry. 'Surely fish is OK?' Fish is a good source of protein and, in oily fish, it can be a good source of essential fats. The trouble with fish is that it is at the top of the food chain again. Big fish eat little fish, they eat smaller ones and so on, down to those that live on tiny marine organisms and plankton.

Regrettably, our industrial and agricultural 'progress' has made our oceans a cesspit of industrial and agricultural pollutants. The run-off from industrial and agricultural production has contaminated every water body on earth and it is now virtually impossible to find uncontaminated fish. They are frequently, if not always, contaminated with toxic heavy metals, including lead and mercury and chemical residues from pesticides and chemical fertilizers that have washed off the land into rivers and seas.

Fish that are farmed in unnatural proximity to one another are often contaminated by chemical feeds, additives to 'colour' their flesh and by eating their own faeces.

So I'm afraid, on balance, Livetetics has to sound a note of caution with fish. It is a very sad reflection of the state of our planet. It is well worth noting that the chemical and agricultural interests that have largely caused this pollution now wish us to trust them with the genetic modification of plants and animals.

I urge that such polluters should not be trusted with a toothbrush! The whole issue of GM food is now riddled with ignorruption, as we have already discussed.

DAIRY PRODUCTS

This is another area that is full of ignorruption. Many people walk into my office convinced that it is essential to eat dairy products. Indeed some force themselves to eat the stuff because their doctors have told them to.

The pushing of dairy products alongside meat as an essential part of the necessary intake for health is quite simply one of the most extraordinary achievements of our 'nutritional' history. It is a monkey pole extraordinaire!

There is no requirement for dairy products at any stage of life unless you are literally starving and there is nothing else available.

Cow's milk, it has to be said, is an excellent food, but only if you happen to be a calf!

The composition of milk, its proteins and fat, is designed to turn a calf into a huge animal in a short space of time. And it can do the same to people. Milk contains proteins that are tough to digest and it carries loads of excess fat. Modern dairy husbandry adds to the deadly cocktail by potentially contaminating it with pesticide residues, hormones and antibiotics. Pasteurization further denatures milk. Even calves fed pasteurized milk do not thrive!

Nursing mothers should stick with nature wherever possible and feed their babies from their own breasts.

I can think of almost nothing more abhorrent than a baby, child or adult sucking from the udder of a cow. It is insanity!

Animal-based foods – meat, dairy and eggs – contain proteins that are tough to digest and produce excess metabolic acids and toxins, thereby stressing your digestive and detoxification systems. They are best avoided altogether or taken in small quantities.

Unfortunately, the 'low calorie' fad which has, potentially, so much to offer by encouraging people to remove junk carbohydrates, has been hijacked to make all carbohydrates 'enemies' and high fat, excess protein animal foods 'good guys'.

I suspect that some food industry interests are at work here. The ascendancy of unwise high protein diets with their potential for kidney damage, mineral leaching, toxic stress and disturbance of metabolic processes, is a great disservice to consumers but a great boon, it must be said, for the meat and dairy industry. Coincidence?

Studies have shown that eaters of animal produce are more significantly at risk from degenerative diseases including heart disease and cancer.

OTHER OPTIONS

The options below provide useful sources of protein and vitamins if they are eaten in limited quantities.

Protein is essential to ensure your metabolic furnace burns brightly. Proteins are tissue and muscle builders. For every pound of muscle gained, your body burns an extra 70 calories an hour. A full spectrum of lean, healthy protein is essential for the building of muscle rather than the deposition of fat.

You don't need much. Livetetic grain and legume consumption will provide all the protein you need but for some the lure of their lifelong conditioning about animal products and 'protein food' is just too hard to pull away from.

SOY

Tofu and tempeh are very versatile foods and can be eaten pretty much with abandon; they are excellent in scrambles, and as part of grilled kebabs or stir-fries. Use herbs and spices to season and add flavour. A portion is in the order of 200g, the best part of a block of tofu or a jar of tempeh.

FISH

Open water (wild) fresh fish is the best kind to include. Avoid farmed fish and raw sushi – these can contain high levels of parasites and may interfere with your digestion. Be careful where you buy fish; it can be hanging around a long time before you get it. Fresh fish barely smells. It starts to get 'fishy' as it turns. Unfortunately, most crustaceans and shellfish live too close to land and so absorb significant amounts of pollutants which we, in turn, ingest when we eat them. They are, therefore, best avoided!

CHICKEN AND EGGS

Take very small portions of chicken or fish but eat what satisfies you. 100g is a piece about the size of your fingers. One egg will do it, two if you must!

Animal products are tough on the digestion. It is best to eat them 20–30 minutes after you have eaten raw foods, fruit and vegetables. Do not eat sugar or refined carbohydrates with meat products, as they can make the digestive process even more acidic and toxic. Avoid eating fruit after eating animal products: leave a space of at least an hour and a half.

Category A – As much as you like			
Tofu	Tempeh		
Category B – 2-3 x week. Moderate			
Salmon	Sardines	Eel	Isolated soy protein
Mackerel	Fresh tuna		powder/shake mix
Category C – up to 2 x week. Limit			
Fresh organic free range chicken	Fresh organic free range eggs	Other fish	Modified/textured soy or veg protein

NOURISHMENT − HELPERS

CRANBERRY

Cranberry juice is full of flavonoids, enzymes and organic acids. The organic acids include malic acid, citric acid and quinic acid and these have an emulsifying effect on fatty deposits in the lymphatic system. Cranberry juice is reported to digest stagnated lymphatic wastes and this is one of the reasons that Livetetics followers report disappearance of cellulite. Cranberry juice must be natural and unsweetened. In a liquid form it is absorbed immediately into the digestive system and rapidly enters the lymphatic system, where it can get on with breaking down and moving on those blocked waste materials. Alternatively, in fact preferably, use a high-quality powder.

CIDER VINEGAR

Having lemon juice or vinegar with meals can lower blood sugar levels by as much as 30 per cent. Livetetics recommends having a glass of lemon water (water with a half or whole fresh squeezed lemon) on rising and having cider vinegar with lunch and evening meal as part of a salad or vegetable dressing.

HERBS AND SPICES

There are a number of herbs and spices that boost your body's ability to metabolize sugar. These include cinnamon, cloves, bay leaf, coriander, cayenne, dry mustard and ginger. Use these herbs alone or in combinations to add flavour and interest to your food. They will do more than make things taste great − they are a fantastic aid to any weight loss effort.

FOOD SUPPLEMENTS – DAILY FOUNDATION

Even with the greatest of care and attention to our diet, we will still benefit from nutritional supplementation. Supplementation with essential vitamins and minerals, in good quantities in bio-available forms, helps ensure we have the best chance of overall nourishment.

It is a sad truth that the lowered nutritional content of modern foods, and the added burden of our polluted world and stressful lives, mean that supplementing your food is now essential.

This is our recommended programme to support your body transformation goals.

Minimum levels

As a minimum, Livetetics recommends you take these food supplements to ensure you get the nutrients you need:

Multinutrient	Multivitamin and mineral – broad spectrum in good forms
Antioxidant	Antioxidant complex (Extra vitamins A, C, E and minerals zinc and selenium)

There is an abundant range of food supplements that deliver nutritional support. Select a high quality multinutrient from a reputable health outlet. Avoid the one-a-day junk supplements advertised on television, you're paying more for advertising and packaging than you are for the nutrients. Some junk multinutrient, sold even in reputable outlets under well-known brand names, contain so little of any vitamin or mineral that the gain you get from taking them is insignificant.

Livetetics does not recommend specific brands. It is better to use a variety. Never buy more than a 30-day supply from any one brand. Different manufacturers use different forms of the nutrients, and different excipients and binders. By rotating your manufacturers, you have the best chance of getting nutrients in a form that will work for you.

Take your multinutrient and antioxidant with a main meal, in the middle of your meal. They are best digested alongside food at the peak of the digestive process.

Some who would attempt to knock Livetetics may accuse me of having some interest in pushing supplements. On the contrary, my wish is for a clean world with food production processes that would mean we get all the nourishment we need from nature. That is how it should be.

Supplementation is a blunt instrument, but our experience is that supplementing food intake with a quality nutritional supplement programme makes a significant difference for most people; particularly those who have not supplemented before.

Obesity, diabetes, heart disease and cancer are all, to a greater or lesser degree, symptoms of imbalance and are directly related to nutritional status. They are altered by the extent to which the body is balanced.

Well-considered supplementation, along with Livetetic nourishment and lifestyle factors, can aid the restoration of balance, help normalize energy and appetite and restore optimum function in key body systems.

Supplements that help other body systems

In addition to your foundation supplements you might like to consider a supplement programme to address any obvious underlying imbalances.

To do this, you should ideally consult with a qualified nutrition practitioner. In most countries finding a competent nutrition practitioner is a bit of a hit and miss affair.

Most doctors know very little about the efficacy of nutrient supplementation and are not trained thoroughly enough to assess underlying functional issues or to look for inter-relationships between body functions, nutrition and the symptoms that you present.

This is changing slowly and there is a move to understanding the impact on health of balance in body systems. In the UK a growing number of doctors study nutrition and environmental effects on health and incorporate these into their practice of medicine. Find one!

There are eight underlying factors that often need assistance from nutritional supplementation in the early stages and these are listed below. If you are philosophically opposed to nutritional supplementation do not fear, you can make enormous strides with adjustments in food intake alone. But, if you are minded to accelerate your progress, it can be beneficial to consider a supplement programme that is targeted at whichever of the following underlying systems is an issue for you.

It is best to focus on one of these at a time. To help prioritize the food adjustments that will have the most rapidly beneficial effect, you can consult with a qualified nutrition practitioner.

If you have any diagnosed condition, are on medication or under a doctor's supervision, be sure to consult with them before you make any substantial change to your food intake or use food supplements targeted at specific health factors.

Specific supplement programme targeted at specific health factors	Hormones
	Energy (blood sugar)
	Detoxification
	Digestion
	Food sensitivity
	Mind and mood
	Heart and circulation
	Immunity

LIFESTYLE

Throughout Livetetics you have been gradually introduced to physical things you can do and hopefully have noticed the difference they can make even while you are reading.

There are some powerful additions you can make to your daily activities that will make a significant positive difference to how you look and feel.

Movement

PULSE-RAISING MOVEMENT 20–30 MINUTES A DAY

Walk, swim, dance or cycle. Just enough to raise your heart rate and increase your breathing. DO NOT get out of breath or risk any discomfort. Maintain a level you feel you could keep up for hours. Enjoy it. Exercise outdoors is better than in the gym.

STRETCH

Gentle stretches before and after you exercise. Take instruction on stretching techniques from a qualified instructor.

RESISTANCE

Load-bearing exercise is essential. Start with little things; carry a basket around the supermarket rather than push a trolley. Carry bags to the car. Get a pair of dumbbells and take instruction in using them. An hour with a personal trainer will repay you a hundred times. Building muscle will dramatically improve your metabolism, fuel your furnace and increase your fat-loss potential. Simple things, big results. Press-ups, sit ups, and pull-ups are amazingly effective.

Resistance exercise is one of the most effective ways to increase bone density and strength, no matter what your age.

Elimination

SKIN BRUSH

Gently brush torso and limbs towards the centre, morning or evening. Start with a soft bristle brush (Body Shop stock good ones) and do this before your shower. Be amazed at how soft your skin becomes! Skin brushing helps clear away debris and toxic wastes through the natural process of skin exfoliation.

10-MINUTE LIE-DOWNS

Lying horizontally flushes your liver with blood and helps it do its job well. Find a way to do this twice a day. In the park or garden, on a bench (under your desk at work!). It is a huge boost to your detoxification system and fat-processing capability.

HOT/COLD SHOWER

Enjoy a warm shower and then, before you get out, alternate hot and cold. Keep it comfortable. Over time you will enjoy this more and more and be able to tolerate quite large shifts in temperature comfortably. Shift 5–10 times for 20–30 seconds a time, and end on cold. This stimulates circulation and aids lymph drainage.

Light and air

SLEEP WITH YOUR WINDOW OPEN

Fresh air at night is the key to a good night's rest. Sleep with the bedroom window open. If it's noisy outside wear earplugs. If you are cold use an extra blanket. Fresh air at night is vital for energy detoxification and a good night's rest.

30-MINUTE WALK OUTSIDE

You should have already covered this with your daily aerobic movement. But try to expose your limbs and face to the elements each day. Easy in the summer, harder to do in the winter, but essential. Fresh air (as fresh as you can get it these days) and sunlight (even if it is through a blanket of cloud) are essential to your system.

Sleep and relaxation

8 HOURS (IDEALLY 10:00PM–06:00 AM)

Try to do this for the next 90 days at least. You need rest. Engage in calming activity 30–40 minutes before bed: restful music, a warm drink, gentle company, soft light, an enjoyable book. Visualize your perfect self as you drift off to sleep.

DON'TS

Avoid negative influences, especially in the evening. Unplug your TV and cancel your paper for 90 days. Find positive and comforting pursuits in their place. Use the opportunity to contact old acquaintances or relations. Take up a favourite hobby, go to concerts, the theatre or enjoy your garden or plants. Take an interest in food preparation or cooking. The world will change little in 90 days but your perception of it will change a great deal! This is one of the most potent things you can do.

Don'ts	Do's
Watch TV	Avoid television and radio
Read rubbish	Avoid newspapers and magazines
Be an ignorrupt	Avoid people or relations who are not supportive

DEGENERATIVE 'FOOD'

D 'foods' put the *die* in *diet*.

Depleted foods
Dysfunctional foods
Drug foods
Depression foods
Dead foods
Damaged foods

These items are all unnecessary in a healthy intake. They are surplus to requirements and are potentially very counterproductive. Commercial imperatives have ensured that the current views on Diet accept these foods in moderation as part of a 'healthy balanced Diet'. The choice is yours.

Livetetics recommends cutting D 'foods' out completely for 90 days to allow your body to renourish and rebalance. Your tastes will shift during this time. You may have some D 'foods' now and then; if you do, enjoy them. Once your internal furnace is burning well, your body should be able to deal with low to moderate amounts of these items. But they are not good, they are not healthy and they do not support the nourishment of your body. They are not food.

These substances, according to Livetetic principles and experience, have a net negative well-being effect. They are so entrenched in Western life and diets because they are cheap, have long shelf-lives and people like them (remember our evolutionary cravings for sweetness, fat and salt). They are potentially very powerful disease promoters and it is likely that within two generations they will be removed from sale to minors. Health warnings similar to those now seen on cigarettes are already being 'tested' on the public by some supermarket chains.

The 90-day exclusion

Removing these substances completely for 90 days is a fascinating exercise. It demands thought before products are dropped into your basket. The best way is to do most of your shopping by staying in the fruit and vegetable section and the aisle containing whole grains and pulses. Get a couple of recipe books. If you focus on the massive variety of real food that you can still enjoy, you will be amazed at the possibilities for truly healthy nourishing food that does not rob you of energy and health. It is going to demand that you prepare food yourself. This is much better than eating leftovers (or the processed food equivalent).

Initially, experience shows that the elimination of Dysfunctional food and ingredients leaves food tasting 'bland' or 'boring'. Don't worry. Within a few short days your natural palate will begin to restore itself and you will, once more, be able to taste your food. The supplement programme will help with this. Most people are deficient in the essential mineral zinc and this undermines your ability to taste food properly.

Refined and processed sugar and other refined carbohydrates

The ultimate dysfunctional ingredient: refined and added sugar is excess to requirements and delivers empty calories, which unbalance the nutrient profile of your intake. All excess carbohydrate turns to fat. Refined sugar is always excess carbohydrate; it is a net negative food because it uses nutrition rather than delivers nutrition. Other refined carbohydrates have similar effects to sugar and a similarly depleted nourishment profile. White bread, cakes, biscuits, white pasta, pizza bases and other low quality junk carbohydrates should ideally be eliminated for 90 days and then, if you have to, reintroduced in very limited quantities.

REQUIREMENT FOR REFINED SUGAR IN A HEALTHY INTAKE: NONE

The maximum amount of sugar tolerable in a healthy intake is the equivalent of 4–5 teaspoons per day or up to five per cent of calories. (The World Health Organization recommends a maximum of ten per cent of calories from sugar. I believe this is a significant overstatement and is driven by the huge weight of lobbying pressure from the sugar peddlers.)

The research my consultancy carried out among 37,053 people in the UK showed that as little as one sugar-based snack would cause adverse reactions in their bodies. After your 90 day elimination, re-introduce these items very sparingly, if at all.

Refined flour products (bread, biscuits, cakes, pizza), white pasta, white rice and other processed carbohydrates should be eliminated for 90 days and then kept to a maximum of one portion every 2–3 days.

If you have a day when you slip on this, because of some event or social occasion, try to go for a brisk walk for an hour as soon as possible after the junk intake. Take an additional multi-nutrient and a supplement containing a good source of chromium.

Expect a lot of people to jump up and down at this recommendation. As we've said before, accepting that refined sugar is not food at all presents a lot of well-educated people with a significant barrier to acceptance. It also threatens the business of the world's largest 'food' manufacturers; among them are many drug companies who peddle sugar waters to children and 'energy' drinks to sports people.

The addition of refined sugars should be shown separately on product labels with calories from refined sugar made clear, and expressed as a percentage of the recommended daily maximum.

Tea, coffee, colas and stimulants

Coffee contains three stimulants. The primary one is caffeine but theobromine and theophylline are also there (even in decaffeinated coffee!). Coffee drinking has been linked with cancer of the pancreas and increased incidence of birth defects. All stimulants increase stress hormones and can unbalance blood sugar. These substances have been associated with pancreatic disturbance, disordered sleep and birth defects. Caffeine can provoke an adrenal response that participates in the adjustment of mood, concentration and feelings of 'energy'. Tea and coffee strip out minerals in the digestive process and reduce your body's ability to get nourishment form food.

Tea has the same effect as coffee but it is less potent. Colas do the same (normally with the inclusion of up to 12 spoons of sugar).

REQUIREMENT FOR TEA, COFFEE AND STIMULANTS IN A HEALTHY INTAKE: NONE

Maximum tolerable: one cup a day, one hour away from a meal and before midday. Maximum 4-5 cups a week.

Note: If you have a day when you take more, then consider taking an additional multimineral and antioxidant.

All products containing caffeine should carry labels showing the milligrams of caffeine delivered per portion and age guidelines on maximum consumption. The 'accepted' maximum in current nutrition thinking is higher than the Livetetic recommendation – mainly due to commercial pressures and dogma. Tea and coffee were early drugs, trafficked around the world by royalty and governments and were important economic components upon which Western economies were built – often in conjunction with slavery.

Tea and coffee should not be consumed by anyone considering having a baby (men and women) or by pregnant or lactating women.

Chocolate and confectionery

Chocolate contains cocoa, which provides significant quantities of the stimulant theobromine. Theobromine acts in much the same way as caffeine. Usually supplied with large doses of sugar this plays havoc with blood sugar and sets off the high/low swings. The lack of nutrients also depletes body stores in processing this lifeless, addictive drug. It's a potential health and well-being killer. All confectionery provides excess refined carbohydrate and empty calories.

Chocolate should be eliminated for 90 days and then incorporated into your refined sugar maximum. Half a standard snack bar a day is the maximum allowable, with a two-day rest each week.

Alcohol

Alcohol comes from letting yeast act on sugar. In the short term, alcohol inhibits the release of reserve glucose from the liver and encourages low blood sugar levels. It can often cause a sharp increase in appetite. Diseases associated with alcohol excess include diabetes, heart disease, cirrhosis, cancer of the liver and gradual deterioration of the brain.

Alcohol is demanding on the liver and reduces the effectiveness of this vital organ. Liver function wasted on alcohol is energy and detoxification capability that could be put to better use.

The much touted 'red herring' of the beneficial effects of alcohol on heart disease (because it has antioxidant properties and can 'thin' the blood) only applies if you are under oxidative stress or have thick, sticky blood. This much publicized 'benefit' of moderate alcohol consumption simply means that it might, from one direction, make already sick people slightly less sick, but it will still stress the liver and make them sick in other ways. There is no doubt to the Livetetic practitioner that, like sugar, any consumption of alcohol has a negative effect on health and well-being.

By all means enjoy some, but it must be respected as the toxic drug that it is. Avoid addiction at all costs.

Maximum consumption of alcohol is two units on a maximum of three days a week. If you are confronted with an occasion where additional consumption is 'essential' then prepare by hydrating fully before the occasion. Drink 1.5 litres of water two hours ahead of the event, and take a high quality B vitamin supplement as well as a supplement giving detoxification support.

Artificial sweeteners

Artificial sweeteners may increase appetite, play havoc with your metabolism and induce an insulin response even though they do not contain any sugar. Because of this artificial sweeteners have the potential to make you put on weight! They are foreign chemicals and have to be detoxified. It is better to allow your liver to perform the more useful task of processing that fat. Some are thought to be neurotoxic. Keep away from these unnatural and potentially dangerous chemicals.

I believe there is significant risk with artificial sweeteners. It seems the research on them is highly unreliable and that the regulatory process may be entirely inadequate to deal with the proliferation of these potentially dangerous and unnecessary chemicals. Read labels and look for artificial sweeteners. Don't eat products that contain them and don't feed them to your children.

They are usually prolific in 'sugar free' and 'diet' products.

Salted foods

Most manufactured and processed foods and snacks contain an excess of salt. Sodium is an essential mineral that was once only found naturally, in small quantities, in the environment. We have evolved to like the taste of salt, and it is now used prolifically as a cheap way of flavouring junk sold as food.

For 90 days avoid any food that contains added salt. Processed, ready meals and take-aways are usually loaded with salt, fat, colourings, preservatives, emulsifiers and low-quality ingredients. They are effectively the same as eating heavily contaminated leftovers and are best left on the shelf. At least for 90 days, dump these cocktails of low-quality contaminated 'food'. After that you will be amazed at how appalling they taste and feel in the mouth and body.

Processed food in all its forms is frequently loaded with salt. This salt is surplus to requirements and messes up the ionic concentration of body fluids. The balance of sodium and potassium in the body is critical to the effective functioning of the cells.

Excess salt is linked to high blood pressure and heart disease. Excess sodium is also potentially a contributor to cancer because of the sodium potassium imbalance it creates.

Excess salt is a killer. Food manufacturers use it because 'taste tests' suggest they should. Your body needs only tiny amounts of salt: processed food is where the excess comes from. Leave it on the shelf, restore your palate and start to learn how delicious natural foods can taste. It will take a little time but it will be worth it!

Avoid packaged, processed, tinned and instant foods for 90 days. You will be amazed at how excessively salty they taste at the end.

Opposite are some tables, taken from a survey report of 37,000 adults I presented at the House of Commons. In them it can be seen that a single sugar-based snack a day halves the likelihood of being in optimum health. Similarly, as little as one cup of tea or coffee a day nearly halves the chance of being optimally well. But low wheat (and dairy) consumers are more than three times as likely to in tip-top condition as are high consumers of refined carbohydrates. Food for thought?

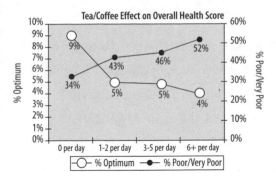

Tea/Coffee Effect on Overall Health Score

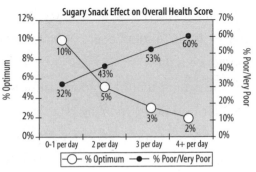

Sugary Snack Effect on Overall Health Score

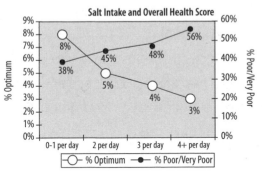

Salt Intake and Overall Health Score

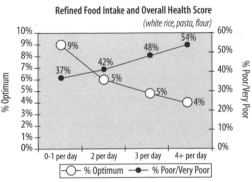

Refined Food Intake and Overall Health Score
(white rice, pasta, flour)

Wheat and dairy

These foods are frequently not tolerated well by people. We find, time and again, that wheat and dairy are implicated in weight gain and ill health, and can produce a range of symptoms, including bloating, flatulence, excess mucus, fluid retention, feeling groggy in the morning, headaches and migraine, eczema, acne or other skin conditions, energy slumps and weight problems. Whatever your sensitivity profile, we recommend eliminating these from your diet as far as possible (preferably completely) for 90 days. Then introduce them again gently (if you must) but don't eat them more than once a day.

The notion that dairy foods are an essential component of any diet is another nutritional monkey pole. It is dogma propagated by an industry that, as with sugar and tea/coffee, used to be controlled by wealthy landowners and governments and was an important part of western economies. It is perfectly possible to get all the minerals you need, including calcium, without relying on cow's milk.

You can expect significant resistance to the idea that you should minimize wheat and dairy products. They are big business and most conventional nutritionists regard dairy as an important 'food group'. Dairy products are not essential and are entirely optional.

Meat

Lean organic meat is a reasonable source of protein and nutrients. Unfortunately it is also a source of unnecessary fat. Modern, non-organic animal husbandry ensures your meat is a cocktail of pesticides, hormones, growth factors, antibiotics and plenty of saturated fat. It is frankly easier to eliminate it and go for the other, much better tolerated and more beneficial sources of nourishment. Go lean and organic if you must add this to your C category protein list.

NOURISHMENT

Daily Foundation

Air	Vital breathing	5 x day
Water	Pure, fresh water	8 x day
Fruit	Fresh, raw or gently cooked fruit	5 x day
Vegetables	Fresh, raw or gently cooked	5 x day
Whole grains	Whole, unrefined grains (variety!)	3-5 x day
Pulses/beans	Fresh cooked beans and pulses (variety!)	3-5 x day
Nuts and seeds	A handful – as a snack or ground/blended	1 x day
Oil	High quality flax oil or oil blend	1-2 x day
Soy/fish/eggs/ chicken	1 portion of soy or fish or chicken or eggs	2-3 x week

Helpers

Cranberry juice	Fresh, unsweetened or quality powder – dilute/dissolve	2 x daily
Cider vinegar	1 tablespoon	Daily
Herbs and Spices	Bay leaf, cayenne, cinnamon, cloves, coriander, cumin, dill, mustard, garlic, ginger, fennel	At least 2 a day, to taste

SUPPLEMENTATION

Added nutrition should support you well – see overleaf for more details. As a minimum take a high quality, high dose multinutrient with vitamins and minerals in easily absorbed forms. You must get the food right first, though. Supplements work best with food; remember, they are supplements and NOT replacements.

Daily foundation

Multinutrient	High quality, broad spectrum multivitamin and mineral	2 x day
Antioxidant	High quality antioxidant complex	1 x day
System support	Primary system support – blood sugar, digestion, detoxification, hormones, food sensitivity, heart and circulation, immunity	1-3 x day

Don't forget that if you are particularly keen to supplement your diet with added nutrients, it is a good idea to go to a specialist for advice. And again, if you have any diagnosed condition or you are under a doctor's supervision, be sure to make them aware of what you are taking.

The 'Do's' below are particularly key to the Livetetic lifestyle. Try to incorporate them into your daily routine and you'll feel the benefit within a couple of weeks.

Do's

Breathing	Vital breathing exercise while walking.	5 x Day
Movement	Constant heart-raising movement 20-30 minutes	Daily
	Stretch	Daily
	Resistance exercises	3 x week
Elimination	Skin brush	Daily
	10-minute lie down	2 x daily
	Hot/cold shower	Daily
Light and Air	Window open	Night
	30-minute walk outside	Daily
Sleep	8 hours (ideally 10:00pm – 06:00 am)	Daily
Relax	Music and meditation 30 mins	Daily

Don'ts

Watch TV	Avoid automatically believing television and radio	Check references
Read rubbish	Avoid automatically believing newspapers and magazines	Check references
Negatives	Avoid arguments and confrontation with people or relations who are not supportive	Avoid confrontation

The ideal is total elimination, but this isn't an ideal world. What is vital to remember is that these foods are surplus to requirement and all are potentially unbalancing. If you have them, enjoy them. But absolute moderation is the key: they are off your path. We recommend total elimination for 90 days while you readjust to your new body. Then, as the cravings subside and you rediscover your natural tastes and preferences, you can delve back into the cess pit – if you really want to!

Dysfunctional Non-Foods

Refined sugar	Including chocolate, sweets, biscuits, cakes	Reduce/Eliminate
Tea and coffee	All caffeinated beverages and stimulant drinks	Reduce/Eliminate
Colas/sodas	Including 'diet' versions	Reduce/Eliminate
Alcohol	All beer, wines and spirits	Reduce/Eliminate
Salt and salt snacks	Added salt, crisps, crackers, nuts	Reduce/Eliminate
Artificial sweeteners	All – including aspartame and saccharin	Reduce/Eliminate

Damaged and Adulterated Foods

Ready meals	Frozen, microwave, canned, packaged	Reduce/Eliminate
Take away	Pizza, Chinese, Indian, etc	Reduce/Eliminate
Restaurant foods	High salt, fat, sugar	Reduce/Eliminate
Microwaved food	Especially processed meals	Reduce/Eliminate

Potential Well-being Blockers

Wheat	Especially in gluten-sensitive people	Reduce/Eliminate
Dairy	Especially if food sensitivities are high	Reduce/Eliminate
Meat	Especially poorly husbanded high fat varieties	Reduce/Eliminate

It takes 6-12 weeks to change your behaviour. Can you go for it for 90 days and see what happens?

Fill in the grid opposite day by day to see how you are doing. Fill in the boxes in the week summary to show how much you achieved in each area. Record your success here over the first two weeks and then turn to pages 288–297 to record your progress over the next ten weeks.

At the end of each week, record how you feel. Look at the areas that went well and think of ways to make it even better the following week.

DAILY LIVETETICS CHECKLIST

Positive Livetetics Elements ADDITIONS		Day 1	Day 2	Day 3	Day 4	Day 5	Day 6	Day 7	Week	
Daily Nourishment		Week 1 2	Week 1 2	Week 1 2	Week 1 2	Week 1 2	Week 1 2	Week 1 2	1	2
Air/Breathing	5 x day									
Water	7 x day									
Fruit	5 x day									
Vegetables	5 x day									
Whole grains	3-5 x day									
Pulses/Beans	3-5 x day									
Nuts and seeds	1 x day									
Oil	1-2 x day									
Helpers										
Cranberry juice	2 x daily									
Cider vinegar	Daily									
Herbs & Spices	Daily									
Supplementation										
Multinutrient	2 x day									
Antioxidant	1 x day									
Lifestyle										
Heart-raising movement	Daily									
Stretching	Daily									
Resistance exercise	Daily									
Elimination										
Skin Brush	Daily									
10-Minute Lie-Downs	2 x Daily									
Hot & Cold Shower	Daily									

Positive Livetetics Elements ADDITIONS		Day 1	Day 2	Day 3	Day 4	Day 5	Day 6	Day 7	Week 1	Week 2
		Week 1 2	Week 1 2	Week 1 2	Week 1 2	Week 1 2	Week 1 2	Week 1 2		
Light & Air										
Window open	Night									
30-Minute outdoor walk	Daily									
Sleep										
8 Hours rest	Daily									
Relax										
Deliberate relaxation 20–30 mins	Daily									

Minimize or Eliminate SUBTRACTIONS	Day 1	Day 2	Day 3	Day 4	Day 5	Day 6	Day 7	Week 1	Week 2
D 'Foods'/Junk									
Sugar									
Tea, Coffee & Stimulants									
Colas/Sodas									
Alcohol									
Salt and salt snacks									
Chocolate and confectionery									
Artificial Sweeteners									
Processed and 'ready' meals									
Take away									
Restaurant foods									
Wheat grains									
Dairy									
Meat									

Don't forget to turn to pages 288–297 to record your achievements for weeks 3–12. How will you feel after 90 days?

LIVE IT – ONE DAY'S MENU

When	Drink	Eat
On rising	Glass of warm lemon water	
Breakfast	Herbal tea or water with fresh juice	Oatmeal made with water or soya milk and grated apple
Mid-morning	Cranberry water	Banana and apricot with handful of nuts and seeds
Lunch	Water with a little fresh juice	Whole-wheat toast with hummus and spinach coleslaw salad
Mid-afternoon	Lemon water or herbal tea	Apricot and pear with a few nuts and/or seeds
Evening meal	Cranberry water	Mixed green salad dressed with oil, lemon and cider vinegar
		Protein of choice flavoured with helper herbs and spices on a bed of lentils and rice with broccoli and/or greens
Evening snack	Herbal tea	Strawberries
On retiring	Water or herbal tea	

Shopping list:

Fruit	Vegetables	Grains	Nuts/Seeds	Pulses/Beans	Protein
One lemon	Spinach	Oatmeal	Mixed nuts and seeds	Lentils	Tofu or
One apple	Coleslaw	Brown rice		Hummus	fish or
One pear	(Carrots,	Bread			chicken or
One banana	cabbage,				eggs
One apricot	onion)				
Strawberries	Broccoli				

Staples: Herbal teas, soy milk, oil blend, herbs and spices

LIVETETICS IN A NUTSHELL

Positive

Nourishment

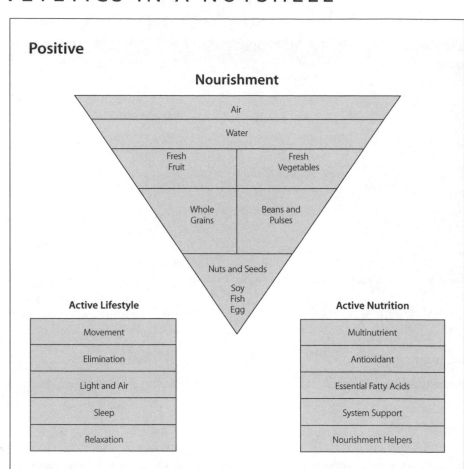

Air

Water

| Fresh Fruit | Fresh Vegetables |
| Whole Grains | Beans and Pulses |

Nuts and Seeds

Soy
Fish
Egg

Active Lifestyle

| Movement |
| Elimination |
| Light and Air |
| Sleep |
| Relaxation |

Active Nutrition

| Multinutrient |
| Antioxidant |
| Essential Fatty Acids |
| System Support |
| Nourishment Helpers |

Negative

Dysfunctional Junk	Adulterated Junk	Potential Blockers
Refined Sugar/ Carbs	Processed Foods	Wheat
Stimulants	Ready Meals	Dairy
Alcohol	Take Away	Meat
Salt	Restaurant Food	
Chemicals		

Below the line in the diagram opposite are aspects of food intake that invariably compromise health and well-being. These are best avoided or eliminated. However this can happen over time. 'Needing' these negative factors is often a result of imbalance and cravings; your 'need' for them declines quite quickly as you restore balance.

As you go through the process, you might like to consult with qualified practitioners in the following practices that can have a powerful effect on re-establishing balance:

- Homoeopathy
- Acupuncture
- Classic osteopathy
- Hypnosis/Neuro-Linguistic Programming

Make sure you get a reference from a satisfied client or get a referral from a practitioner you trust and ensure your practitioner is registered with a reputable body.

Making it happen

W hat do you want? If you are full of energy, feel fantastic, look great, can cope with everything life throws at you, are thrilled to be alive, are completely healthy and fulfilled in every area of your life then don't bother with Livetetics. What you are already doing is working for you.

If your life is perfect, if you are happy with the way you look and feel and you don't want things to be any better, then I would recommend you stay as you are. Things are already working for you. You could try the 90-day Livetetic test just to see what happens. It might be interesting to see how much better things could be.

For the rest of us the 90-day programme is a must. It makes for re-nourishment, rebalancing and a great foundation for optimal well-being. It provides an escape route from the nutritional rut that most of us find ourselves in.

It can be very easy. Remember …

LITTLE BY LITTLE – FOCUS ON THE ADDITIONS

Incremental change can be a good way to go about it. Focus day by day on the additions: the 'Do's'. It is much easier to make the additions than to remove the junk. You will find that by doing so you start to crave the junk less and to like the alternatives more. Going for the whole programme from day one is too much for most people. We recommend introducing the 'Do's' two or three at a time over a 2–3 day period, then add some more. Once you are doing it all, then you can start on the eliminations.

SUSTAINABLE CHANGE

Make the changes in a way that you can sustain them. Livetetics is not a DIEt, it is a way of life. Start as you mean to carry on. Do the things that are easiest for you first. For some it is the breathing, for others the water, for another the supplements. Whatever component you choose to add first, you will find it has a cascading effect that makes it easier to do the rest.

Remember that if you keep doing what you have always done, you will keep getting what you've always got. If you want a different result, try a different behaviour.

Incremental sustainable change; this is what Livetetics is about.

DO IT NOW – BECAUSE NOW IS WHEN YOUR FUTURE BEGINS

Start with your next breath. Go ahead and take ten vital breaths and tick the first box. It's that simple. Focus on the additions. Let the subtractions take care of themselves as you get back into balance. You don't even have to think about them; there is no willpower required, no denial, no guilt, no counting. Picture yourself in 90 days' time.

Just focus on the additions. Start with the easy ones: breathe, drink water, move. Add some fruit and vegetables. Add some grains. Add the beans and pulses. Take a quality multivitamin.

It isn't anything other than very easy.

Do it at your own pace. Focus on the things you like. Find your own hunger and satisfaction levels. Be kind to yourself when you reach for the junk you've become conditioned to go for.

KEEPING IT GOING

Make a weekly picture of your destiny. Make it clearly. Make it big and bright and bold. Really associate with the you that you are working towards. Make it fun. Make a deliberate decision before every sip or bite. What am I hungry for?

Am I hungry?

What is my destiny?

Where will this decision take me?

Enjoy the process. Use your hunger scale and play with your beliefs. Check your references all the time. Read the labels and make positive decisions about what you want to put in your mouth.

We live, fortunately for us, in a free world. No one forces us to put anything in our mouths. We choose. And with every breath, every sip every bite, we choose our destiny. It is our choice.

Choose: a lean healthy body or a fat, sagging mess?

Choose: happiness and feeling in control or misery and depression?

Choose: the decisions start now. Think. Breathe. Eat. Move.

What, how and how much is up to you. No one else.

ANTIDOTES – THINK THROUGH A 'BLOW-OUT'

Be kind to yourself. If you slip, just dust yourself off and get on with it. No need to feel guilty when you fall and scrape your knee. Your body is magical; it will forgive a certain amount of abuse. But take care, the junk is addictive and it can be a slippery slope. Respect it.

Every moment is an opportunity to learn about what does and does not work. There will be times when you just can't be bothered and you trip up. When you do, work out where that moment came from, how the decision was made, think about what to do the next time and then pick yourself up and start again.

Every moment presents another chance for perfection. There are no failures, only opportunities to discover what didn't work as well as it should and to find another way.

YOUR PAST DOES NOT EQUAL YOUR FUTURE

Where you have been has nothing to do with where you are going. What you used to be is nothing to do with what you decide to be today.

If, in the past you have not been successful that is no indication of your potential. Today is a new day and today you are a new you.

What will happen if you don't change? Make a picture of your negative destiny. If you keep doing what you're doing then where are you headed? If you keep doing what you've always done you'll keep getting what you've always got.

Change or stay the same?

Your choice.

CREATE YOUR COMPELLING FUTURE

Build a detailed picture of your future. Spend a minute making this picture in the morning before you get out of bed. Do the same as you drift off to sleep at night. Always focus on what you are doing well and make a small improvement every day. Do this in addition to your weekly written summary.

What others look like, what others deem 'good looking', what others might think about you is completely irrelevant. Beauty, looks, attractiveness are far more than shape and size and colour. It is much more about a radiation of life, vitality and well-being. Being truly well, feeling truly great will allow you to express your utter beauty and laugh at the shallow, lowest common denominator ideals postulated by those who select the fashion of the day. That is why your image of your perfect self must be based on you and not on some idea of someone else or some group that you have been told to admire because they are 'glamorous' or 'cool' or 'fashionable' or 'hard' or 'smart', according to the transient ideals of a magazine editor, advertising creative or television producer.

The references all around you, by which you judge your own beauty, are not relevant to you. Because you are what you are. Your body is your body. What you must do is aspire to your own perfection and then achieve it. Perfection – by your own standards – is your true destiny. Your perfection is a much greater and deeper thing than the flimsy, shallow images that are fed to you each day.

REMOVE YOUR LIMITING BELIEFS

On the pages opposite and over, write down all the reasons why you can't or won't do this – there's an expample there to start you off. Then write down the exact opposites and adopt the opposites as your new beliefs. Add them to the good resources you already have and start to act as that new person. Change is a heartbeat away. With every heartbeat you get another chance to change.

Reasons why I can't do this	Reasons why I can and must do this
Example: This is impractical. I haven't got time to do all of these things.	I can make this easy and fun, and if I really think about it I can make time.

Reasons why I can't do this	Reasons why I can and must do this

EAT ONLY WHEN YOU ARE HUNGRY

Remember also your hunger scale. Only eat when you are genuinely hungry. Avoid and ignore the non-hunger cues: events, time of day, parties, friends, work breaks, boredom, upsets and so. Focus on what you really need. If it isn't food, then don't eat.

Picture your compelling future. See the path that takes you there. Ask, 'Am I hungry?' Check. Where are you on the hunger scale? If you are hungry, then think about what you really want to eat. What does my body want to help it move to my future? Imagine eating whatever it is and think about how you will feel afterwards. Remember, if that chocolate bar immediately jutted out as fat on your bottom, would you eat it? Ask, 'Is this food going to clog me or cleanse me?'

FOCUS ON WHAT YOU WANT, NOT WHAT YOU DON'T WANT

If you focus on what you don't want, then that is probably what you'll get as you are spending your time thinking about that, and not, therefore, focusing on, and working to achieve, what it is you truly want. Imagine yourself achieving your goals in great detail. See yourself winning gold. You are, after all a natural born winner. One of half a million who won the race. You must see yourself achieving what you want. The following section goes into this in more detail.

> *As Buddha is known to have said:*
> *'Believe nothing because it is written in books.*
> *Believe nothing because wise men say it is so.*
> *Believe nothing because it is religious doctrine.*
> *Believe it only because you know it yourself to be true.'*

GET SPECIFIC ABOUT WHAT YOU WANT

Answer the questions below and describe in detail, on paper, what it is you want. Describe in glorious detail the vision you have of the perfect you and then work towards it with every decision you make. With every thing you do, don't do, say, don't say, eat, don't eat, think, don't think – everything MUST drive towards your vision.

> What is it I am really after?
> How will I feel?
> How will people react to me?
> How will I behave?
> What will people think of me?
> What will I think about myself?
> What will I do?
> What will I become?

FOCUS ON THE ADDITIONS

It is much easier to add things to what you do rather than take things away. Focus on the additions to make life easier. Add the water, add the fruit, add the vegetables, add the grains, add the beans and pulses, add the nuts and seeds, add the oil, add the supplement/s. Then the subtractions will take care of themselves. Focus on what you can have and let the rubbish take care of itself.

DON'T 'SHOULD' ALL OVER YOURSELF

If you are going to get what you want there are some things you MUST do. Look at the 'musts' opposite:

> How **must** you feel?
>
> How **must** you treat your body?
>
> What **must** you eat?
>
> How much **must** you exercise?
>
> How clear **must** you make your goals?

'Should' is useless.

THERE IS NO SUCH THING AS FAILURE

You cannot fail. You can only learn about something that doesn't work. Always congratulate yourself when you 'fall over'. Treat yourself gently. Enjoy life. When you eat or live in an inappropriate way, one snack, one meal, one day, one crazy weekend, one holiday, one particularly stressful period, just take stock and learn.

> Congratulate yourself for knowing it wasn't the best thing to do
>
> Forgive yourself
>
> Examine what happened
>
> Plan for next time
>
> Practise your plan in your mind

BRING YOURSELF TO THRESHOLD – NOW

Don't be the frog in the gradually heated pan of water. Notice how hot it is and get out NOW!

You are on your way. You have your manual. It is simple, it is obvious and you can do it.

Enjoy yourself. Enjoy Livetetics!

Start young, stay healthy: Livetetics and children

et's save our children from following our habits just because we never thought to question them for ourselves. The situation with the health of our children is getting pretty serious.

Our children are in poor health

- 20 per cent of children are overweight and one in ten are obese
- Up to a fifth of children have eczema
- Treatment for asthma has doubled in the last ten years
- Hyperactivity (ADHD) is one of the biggest growth areas of medicine
- One in ten children are on prescribed medication at any time
- Up to 40 per cent of children have sluggish bowels with less than one healthy movement a day
- Current statistics show that the majority of our children will die with a chronic, degenerative disease. Cancer, heart disease or diabetes are all significantly, if not entirely, influenced by what they eat and don't eat.

Our children are eating too much junk

The foods commonly eaten by our children are of poor nutritional value:

- 80 per cent of young ones are eating white bread, savoury snacks, crisps, biscuits and chocolate confectionery although none of these are necessary in a healthy diet.
- Three quarters of children drink highly sugared, carbonated soft drinks, totally unnecessary in a healthy diet.
- 34 per cent of children's diets are made up of unnecessary fat

Our children are missing out on key micronutrients

A 1995 MAFF (now the Department for Environment, Food and Rural Affairs) National Diet and Nutrition survey among children aged 1.5-4.5 years showed deficient intakes of a range of essential nutrients. These are summarized opposite.

Nutrient	% deficient	Needed for	Possible signs of deficiency
Zinc	89 per cent	Immunity, brain function, growth, sight, taste and smell	Frequent and/or lingering infections, poor wound healing, skin disorders, white marks on nails, behavioural problems, suboptimal growth
Iron	57 per cent	Carrying oxygen around the body and energy production	Listlessness, fatigue, irritability, pale skin, cracking of lips and tongue, generally feeling poorly, vertical ridges on nails
Iodine	46 per cent	Thyroid function, metabolism, skin, hair and nails, brain development	Depressed growth, listlessness, sluggish behaviour, mental problems
Magnesium	34 per cent	Healthy bones, heart function, nerve impulses, tooth enamel	Muscle contractions, convulsions, irritability, tantrums, skin problems
Vitamin C	34 per cent	Healthy gums and teeth, growth, tissue repair and wound healing	Easy bruising, nosebleeds, frequent infections, weakness, tiredness, paleness, hangnails
Calcium	24 per cent	Bones and teeth, muscle and nerve function, blood clotting	Muscle cramps, muscle contractions, weak bones, poor teeth, dry or brittle nails

Many child disorders are linked to diet

The appalling diets among our children are likely to be a fundamental cause of childhood disorders and illness. If current poor nutrition continues the prognosis is an increase in chronic degenerative disease among adults (heart disease, diabetes, cancer) and a continuation in the proliferation of childhood disorders including asthma, hyperactivity (ADHD), behavioural problems, obesity, and skin problems.

Demonstrations of variation in nutritional quality

HEALTHY SNACK VERSUS JUNK SNACK

Consider the nutritional components delivered to a child by two different snacks as described below:

Healthy snack	Junk snack
Apple	Chocolate bar
Handful of raisins and sunflower seeds	Packet of crisps
Glass of fresh orange juice	Carton of sugary 'fruit' drink

The tables opposite demonstrate the huge variation in quality of different foods. The healthy snack is considerably more beneficial than the junk snack. Consumer awareness and perception of this enormous difference should be greatly improved.

Some foods are very clearly more nourishing than others. A basic nutritional analysis of these two snacks over the next three pages shows virtually the same overall calorie delivery but with a markedly superior macro- and micro-nutrition profile. The healthy snack offers more vitamins, more minerals and far less fat and salt.

It can be seen how the junk snack compromises optimum nutrition by delivering empty calories, excess fat and excess salt. It is a nutritionally inferior option and is a potential contributor to deteriorating child health.

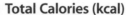

Total Calories (kcal)

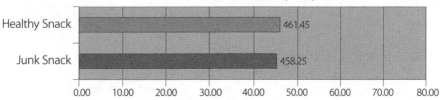

Saturated Fat (g)

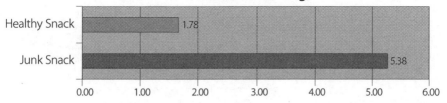

Salt (mg)

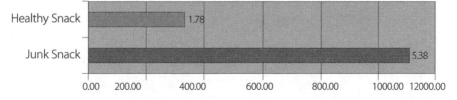

Processed Sugars (g)

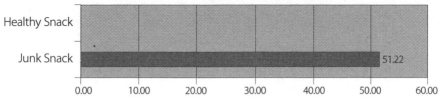

Protein (g)

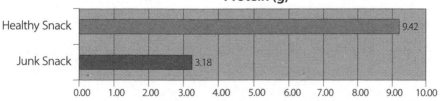

Healthy Snack
Junk Snack

Calcium

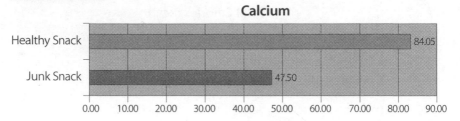

Magnesium

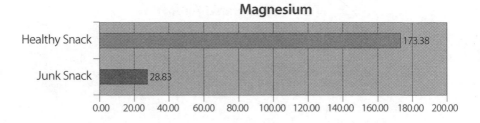

Iron

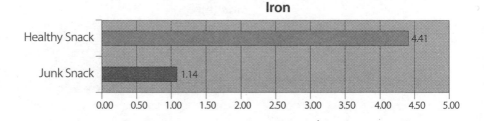

Zinc

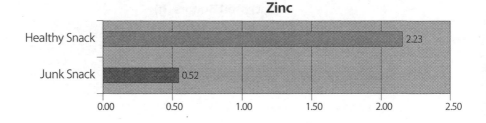

Selenium

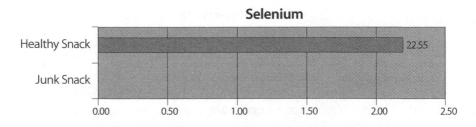

Vitamin A

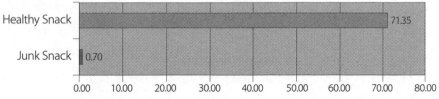

Healthy Snack — 71.35
Junk Snack — 0.70

Vitamin E

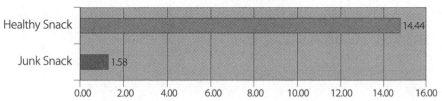

Healthy Snack — 14.44
Junk Snack — 1.58

Folate

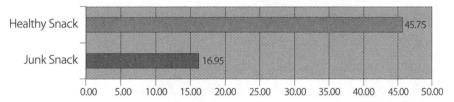

Healthy Snack — 45.75
Junk Snack — 16.95

Vitamin C

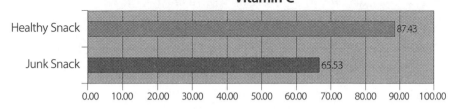

Healthy Snack — 87.43
Junk Snack — 65.53

Iodine

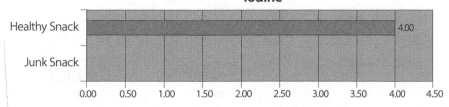

Healthy Snack — 4.00
Junk Snack —

Beware the sugar pushers

'Would you give your child a cup of tea with ten spoons of sugar in it?'

I recently spent a day in three boroughs of south west London asking mothers basic questions about the composition of foods. In particular, they were asked to estimate, in terms of level teaspoons, the amount of sugar to be found in products. From this very qualitative and anecdotal survey of just over 50 people, it was discovered that only one had any idea about the sugar content of common 'snack foods' for children. Everyone interviewed had just bought a junk snack for a child. All had given an unequivocal 'NO' to the above question.

What is obvious is that the contents of food products are not clear from the 'Nutrition Information' on the packet. Calories, grams, per cent, RDA etc, mean very little to people. When this information is put into more understandable language it provides what proved to be a rather shocking insight to all of the parents interviewed.

Parents consistently underestimate what they are giving to children and the average estimates do not reflect immediate perceptions. Once asked to think about it, parents gradually increased their estimates as they did so.

This is a stark indication of the failing of government guidelines, nutrition labelling and consumer awareness. Excess calorie intake is the fundamental root of weight gain and obesity. Knowing how much refined sugar is in a food is an absolute requirement if healthy choices are to be made.

A review of two Sunday morning commercial channels logged over 40 minutes of sugar-pushing advertising to children, with no guidance on healthy intakes, sugar content or healthy alternatives.

Junk Food Content Survey Level teaspoon of sugar = 4.0 grams

Category	Product	Type	Weight/size	Actual spoons of sugar in product	Average estimate of parents
Soft drink	Fortified sports drink	1 Bottle	380.0 ml	**17.0**	5.0
Soft drink	Orange flavour 'fruit' juice	330ml Serving	330.0 ml	**15.7**	3.0
Soft Drink	Chocolate bar inspired drink	Carton	190.0 g	**10.8**	4.0
Soft Drink	Blackcurrant juice drink	Carton	288.0 ml	**10.1**	4.0
Soft Drink	Big name brand cola	1 Can	330.0 ml	**8.7**	5.0
Confectionery	Child's sweets mix	Child Pack	40.5 g	**8.7**	2.0
Confectionery	Baby jellies	Child Pack	40.0 g	**8.0**	3.0
Confectionery	Wine gums	1 Roll	52.0 g	**5.5**	3.0
Confectionery	Popular chocolate bar	85 g Bar	85.0 g	**11.5**	5.0
Confectionery	'Leisure' chocolate bar	Regular Bar	65.0 g	**11.4**	5.0
Confectionery	Finger-shaped fudge bar	Child Bar	26.5 g	**4.5**	3.0
Confectionery	Chocolate bar with light centre	Child Bar	26.0 g	**4.4**	2.0
Confectionery	Round-shaped chocolate drops	Child Pack	32.0 g	**4.3**	2.0
Confectionery	Star-shaped chocolates	Child Pack	32.0 g	**4.3**	2.0
Confectionery	White chocolate	Child Bar	25.0 g	**3.4**	2.0

The table above is a roll-call of shame. Listed are some common soft drink and confectionery junk snacks. The last two columns are the most revealing. Compare what the parents thought the snacks had in terms of sugar content, to the actual sugar content. Not only is the actual sugar content almost obscenely high, but there is a huge difference in the parents' expectations of the sugar content, and the actual sugar content.

Start looking at labels (the ones that are clear, anyway) and see just how much sugar is put into everyday foodstuffs – savoury foods included. It is pretty alarming.

What a difference a menu makes

All of the following diets are actual examples from food logs presented to my network of practitioners. The 'good' menu is a post-consultation menu that was followed with high compliance for 90 days and resulted in significant behavioural improvement, weight loss and enhanced energy for Chris, a 5-year-old boy who was not doing at all well at school. Initially, his mother was very concerned that Chris wouldn't take to diet modifications but, with perseverance, he has made positive changes and now prefers more nutritious foods over junk.

Component	'Good' Menu	'Typical' Menu	'Junk' Menu
Breakfast	Porridge with seed milk and banana. Orange juice	Puffed rice with milk. White toast. Squash	Blackcurrant juice, chocolate bar
Snack	Raisins and Sunflower seeds. Water with a little fresh juice	Biscuit. Milk	Biscuit
Lunch	Tuna sandwich with cherry tomatoes and cucumber. Glass of soya milk	Pork sausages, mashed potato, baked beans. Sponge pudding and custard.	Sausage and oven chips. Ice cream
Snack	Apple. Water with a little fresh juice	Crisps and cola	Crisps and cola
Tea/Dinner	Two clementines. Some grapes. Chicken breast with brown rice, broccoli and green beans	Tinned spaghetti, oven chips, peas. Chocolate bar	Pizza. Chocolate biscuits

The nutritional analysis of these real menus opposite shows that not all calories are equal. The 'typical' menu, in spite of providing significantly more calories than the 'good' menu, does not deliver nearly as much of the key minerals and is much higher in fat. The 'junk' menu provides high fat and even lower levels of minerals.

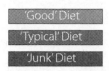

Total Calories (kcal)

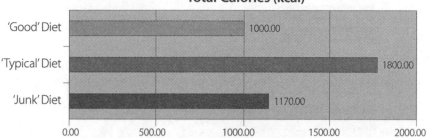

'Good' Diet	1000.00
'Typical' Diet	1800.00
'Junk' Diet	1170.00

0.00   500.00   1000.00   1500.00   2000.00

Saturated Fat (g)

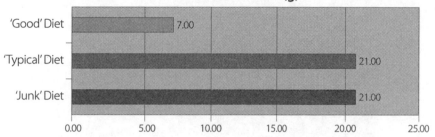

'Good' Diet	7.00
'Typical' Diet	21.00
'Junk' Diet	21.00

0.00   5.00   10.00   15.00   20.00   25.00

Calcium

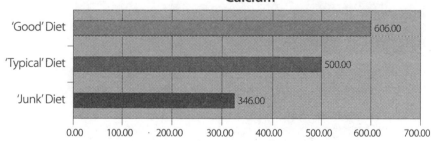

'Good' Diet	606.00
'Typical' Diet	500.00
'Junk' Diet	346.00

0.00   100.00   200.00   300.00   400.00   500.00   600.00   700.00

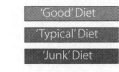

Vitamin C

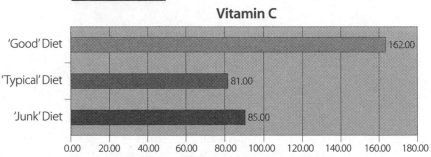

'Good' Diet — 162.00
'Typical' Diet — 81.00
'Junk' Diet — 85.00

0.00 20.00 40.00 60.00 80.00 100.00 120.00 140.00 160.00 180.00

Zinc

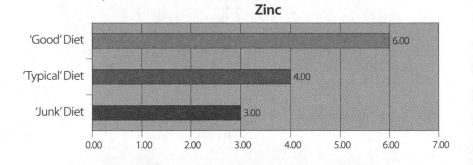

'Good' Diet — 6.00
'Typical' Diet — 4.00
'Junk' Diet — 3.00

0.00 1.00 2.00 3.00 4.00 5.00 6.00 7.00

Selenium

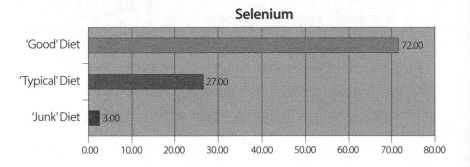

'Good' Diet — 72.00
'Typical' Diet — 27.00
'Junk' Diet — 3.00

0.00 10.00 20.00 30.00 40.00 50.00 60.00 70.00 80.00

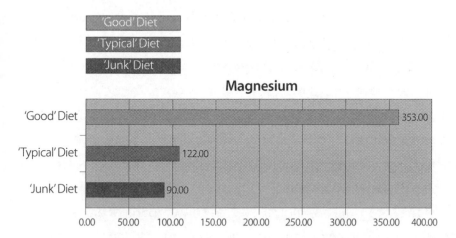

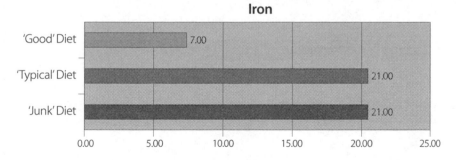

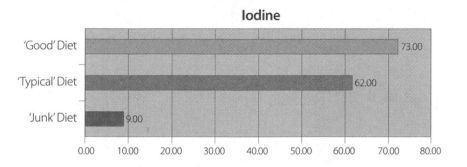

Kill them with love

Ignorruption rules. I have a client whose child attends a school in my county. It is a very good school, an independent junior school for 4 to 11-year-olds, parents pay a great deal of money to send their children there. It has a philosophy of optimizing the potential of the child. It is run by good people, with love and powerful, good intentions. The school has well-founded principles and it acknowledges the importance of self-respect, love and understanding. The school has standards. It is forbidden to drink alcohol or smoke tobacco on the grounds or in the buildings – for pupils, teachers, workmen or anyone.

Yet the school unknowingly allows the consumption of drugs and junk. The teachers drink coffee and eat chocolate biscuits. Indeed, it provides drugs every day to the children in its care.

Here is a typical week's menu:

Monday	Tuesday	Wednesday	Thursday	Friday
SAUSAGE ROLLS	CHICKEN IN GRAVY	SAVOURY MINCE	SLICED ROAST PORK AND GRAVY	FISH CAKE
VEGE NUGGETS	VEGE SAUSAGES	VEGETABLE PIE	MACARONI CHEESE	VEGETABLE SAUSAGE TOAD
JACKET WEDGES	BRAISED RICE	PARSLEY POTATOES	ROAST POTATOES	CHIPPED POTATOES
SWEETCORN	CUCUMBER STIX	SAVOY CABBAGE	BROCCOLI FLORETS	GARDEN PEAS
BAKEWELL TART	SHORT BREAD	JAM SPONGE	FRUIT JELLY AND ICE CREAM	FAIRY CAKE
Fresh Fruit available	Fresh Fruit available	Fresh Fruit available	Fresh Fruit available	Fresh Fruit available

It is a menu riddled with salt and sugar and fat and depleted food. Virtually no whole foods, practically no raw or fresh foods and a mass of highly refined fast- releasing sugars. This is no way to nourish a child. The caterer's use of the 'fresh fruit available' is a catch-all. This is a menu for children aged 4 to 11 years. What chance do they have of making the right decision? Especially if they have already had a sweet biscuit at break that has set up a negative sugar cascade and predisposed their systems towards a poor food selection.

But the scary thing is that the dieticians at the school's catering company hold up the government minimum guidelines (woolly and ineffective though they are) and say that they 'meet the government guidelines'. And when challenged on the issue of sugared dessert the dinner ladies' manager responds, 'Oh, but children need the energy. For some the fruit isn't enough.'

It is criminal. That we should so malnourish a child, so corrupt a palate, so compromise perfection and do it in the name of education, love and understanding. That this abuse meets government guidelines is even more reprehensible.

No one in that school is responsible for this child abuse. They are doing their best with the information, knowledge and expertise they have available. Ignorruption is to blame.

Self-reliance and self-reference is the grand thing. Parents and teachers need to look much deeper than the government guidelines. There are lives at stake.

Key nutrients:
what they do and where
to get them

In various places in this book, specific nutrients and their roles have been mentioned. Just in case you want to pay special attention to getting enough of any specific vitamin or mineral, here is a useful list of sources.

Vitamin A

Sources
Yellow and red vegetables and fruit, dark green vegetables Fish liver oil, liver, margarine, butter, cheese, eggs

Functions	Signs linked with possible deficiency
• Eyesight and night vision	• Mouth ulcers
• Maintenance of skin bones and mucous membranes	• Poor night vision
• Protein synthesis	• Diarrhoea
• Immune system	• Acne
• Cancer inhibition	• Frequent colds or infections
• Growth	• Dry flaky skin
• Reproduction	• Dandruff
	• Thrush or cystitis

Vitamin D

Sources
Formed by action of sunlight on skin (acting on precursor 7-dehydrocholesterol) Oily fish, milk, egg yolk, animal livers, fish

Functions	Signs linked with possible deficiency
• Promotes absorption of calcium and phosphate (thyroid/parathyroid function)	• Rheumatism or arthritis
• Promotes calcium release for distribution and mineral uptake by bones	• Tooth decay
• Nerve function	• Hair loss
• Assists absorption of vitamin A	• Excessive sweating
	• Muscle cramps or spasms
	• Joint pain or stiffness
	• Lack of energy

Vitamin E

Wheat-germ oil, oils of nuts and seeds, vegetables (especially green), legumes, lettuce, peanuts, whole-wheat and wheat sprouts
Fish, eggs, butter

Functions	Signs linked with possible deficiency
• Antioxidant/protects other nutrients	• Lack of sex drive/infertility
• Protects cardiovascular system	• Exhaustion after light exercise
• Reduces muscle requirement of muscles	• Easy bruising
• Improves resistance to infection	• Slow wound healing
• Skin growth and repair	• Varicose veins
• Sex organ function	• Loss of muscle tone

Vitamin C

Sources

Fruit, citrus, blackcurrants, vegetables, potatoes, tomatoes, cabbage family, salad vegetables, sprouted beans, seeds.

Functions	Signs linked with possible deficiency
• Antioxidant/protects other nutrients	• Frequent colds
• Prevents cellular damage	• Lack of energy
• Detoxifies heavy metals	• Frequent infections
• Protects from cancer-causing agents	• Bleeding or tender gums
• Makes collagen – keeps skin, bones, joints and arteries healthy	• Easy bruising
• Enhances wound healing	• Nose bleeds
• Enhances immune system	• Slow wound healing
• Reduces cholesterol levels	• Red pimples on the skin
• Aids iron absorption	
• Produces anti-stress hormones	
• Brain and nerve function	
• Activates folic acid	

Vitamin B1

Sources

Brown rice, wheat-germ, nuts, legumes, soya beans, whole grains, potatoes, dried brewer's yeast, yeast extract
Poultry, meat, milk

Functions	Signs linked with possible deficiency
• Conversion of glucose to energy	• Tender muscles
• Involved in protein metabolism	• Eye pains
• Brain function (production of acetylcholine)	• Irritability
• Needed for efficient digestion	• Poor concentration
	• 'Prickly' legs
	• Poor memory
	• Stomach pains
	• Constipation
	• Tingling hands
	• Rapid heart beat

Vitamin B2

Sources

Yeast extract, brewer's yeast, whole grains, cereal, wheat-germ, legumes, soya beans, green vegetables, avocado pears, nuts, potatoes.
Dairy, liver, eggs

Functions	Signs linked with possible deficiency
• Conversion of fats, sugars and protein to energy	• Burning or gritty eyes
• Repair and maintenance of body tissues	• Sensitivity to bright lights
• Regulation of body acidity (continued...)	• Sore tongue
• Helps eyesight	• Cataracts
• Formation of healthy skin, hair and nails	• Dull or oily hair
	• Eczema or dermatitis
	• Split nails
	• Cracked lips

Vitamin B3

Sources

Yeast extract, brewer's yeast, wheat bran, cereals and whole grains (especially sprouting grains), peanuts
Meat (especially poultry)

Functions	Signs linked with possible deficiency
• Participates in cell respiration	• Diarrhoea
• Produces energy from sugars, fats and protein	• Insomnia
• Production of serotonin – crucial to brain function	• Headaches or migraines
• Helps maintain normal blood sugar levels	• Poor memory
• Helps circulatory system	• Anxiety or tension
• Lowers cholesterol and triglyceride levels	• Depression and lack of energy
• Elevates HDLs (good cholesterol)	• Irritability
• Maintains healthy skin, nerves, brain, tongue and digestive system	• Bleeding or tender gums
• Involved in synthesis of sex hormones	• Acne

Vitamin B5

Sources

All plant and animal tissue (See other B vitamin sources)

Functions	Signs linked with possible deficiency
• Involved in energy production	• Muscle tremors or cramps
• Production of anti-stress hormones	• Apathy
• Control of fat metabolism	• Poor concentration
• Formation of antibodies	• Burning feet or tender heels
• Maintenance of healthy nerves	• Nausea or vomiting
• Maintains health of skin and hair	• Lack of energy
	• Exhaustion after light exercise
	• Anxiety or tension
	• Teeth grinding

Vitamin B6

Sources

Brewer's yeast, wheat bran, cereals, green vegetables, yeast extract, soya flour, legumes, nuts, brown rice, peanuts, potatoes
Animal and dairy produce

Functions	Signs linked with possible deficiency
• Involved in amino acid metabolism	• Infrequent dream recall
• Synthesis of brain chemicals	• Water retention
• Vital for blood formation	• Tingling hands
• Energy production	• Depression or nervousness
• EFA metabolism	• Irritability
• Anti depressant, anti-allergy function	• Muscle tremors or cramps
	• Lack of energy
	• Flaky skin

Vitamin B12

Sources

Spirulina algae (analogue of B12 – may not function in humans). Some yeast products. Formed by bacteria.
Meat, fish, dairy

Functions	Signs linked with possible deficiency
• Protein, fat and carbohydrate metabolism	• Poor hair condition
• Production of red blood cells	• Eczema or dermatitis
• Synthesis of DNA	• Mouth very sensitive to hot or cold
• Production of nerve insulation	• Irritability
• Energy production	• Anxiety or tension
• Detoxification of cyanide in food and tobacco	• Lack of energy
	• Constipation
	• Tender or sore muscles
	• Pale skin

Folic Acid

Sources

Brewer's yeast, soya flour, wheat germ/bran, nuts, cereals, green leafy vegetables, whole grains, pulses, brown rice
Liver, eggs

Functions	Signs linked with possible deficiency
• Involved in protein synthesis	• Eczema
• Blood formation	• Cracked lips
• Builds immunity in newborn infants	• Prematurely greying hair
• Function of nervous system	• Anxiety or tension
	• Poor memory
	• Lack of energy
	• Depression
	• Poor appetite
	• Stomach pains

Biotin

Sources

All plant tissues – especially yeasts, and whole grains
All animal tissue – especially liver, kidney, egg yolk, fish and milk

Functions	Signs linked with possible deficiency
• Involved in metabolism of proteins, fats and carbohydrates	• Dry skin
• Maintaining a healthy skin and hair	• Poor hair condition
• Sweat glands	• Prematurely greying hair
• Nerves, bone marrow and sex glands	• Tender or sore muscles
	• Poor appetite or nausea
	• Eczema or dermatitis

Essential Fatty Acids – Linoleic Acid and GLA

Sources
Seed and nut oils – especially flax, evening primrose, safflower

Functions	Signs linked with possible deficiency
• Production of life energy from food	• Dry rough skin
• Growth vitality and mental state	• Dry eyes
• Facilitate energy production	• Frequent infections
• Structural part of all cell membranes	• Poor memory
• Shorten recovery time for fatigued muscles	• Loss of hair or dandruff
• Procurers of prostaglandins	• Excessive thirst
	• Poor wound healing
	• PMS or breast pain
	• Infertility

Calcium

Sources
Seeds, nuts, root vegetables - almonds, brewer's yeast, parsley, pumpkin seeds, cooked dried beans, whole wheat Milk, cheese

Functions	Signs linked with possible deficiency
• Component of bones and teeth	• Muscle cramps or tremors
• Nerve transmission	• Childhood 'growing' pains
• Needed for muscle action	• Dizziness or poor sense of balance
• Buffers excess acidity	• Fits or convulsions
• Aids blood clotting	• Sore knees
• Controls cholesterol levels	

Magnesium

Sources

Green leafy vegetables, nuts and seeds – wheat-germ, almonds, cashews, brewer's yeast, buckwheat flour, brazil nuts, peanuts, pecan nuts, cooked beans, garlic, raisins, peas, potato skin

Functions	Signs linked with possible deficiency
• Component in bones and teeth	• Muscle tremors or spasms
• Relaxes muscles	• Muscle weakness
• Stabilizes heartbeat and maintains cardiovascular health	• Insomnia or nervousness
• Transmits nerve impulses	• High blood pressure
	• Irregular heartbeat
	• Constipation
	• Fits or convulsions
	• Sore knees

Iron

Sources

Green leafy vegetables, dried fruits, whole grains, beans, lentils
Fish and meat

Functions	Signs linked with possible deficiency
• Component of haemoglobin – transports oxygen to and from cells	• Pale skin
• Component of SOD (Superoxide dismutase – protects against free radicals)	• Sore tongue
• Part of electron transport chain – energy production	• Fatigue or listlessness
	• Loss of appetite or nausea
	• Heavy periods or blood loss

Zinc

Whole foods, whole grains, nuts, seeds,
Fish and meat

Functions	Signs linked with possible deficiency
• Component of 100+ enzymes	• Poor sense of taste or smell
• Component of RNA/DNA	• White marks on more than two finger nails
• Vital for growth and healing	• Frequent infections
• Metabolism of pituitary adrenals, ovaries, testes	• Stretch marks
• Needed for nervous system and brain	• Poor appetite
• Aids bone and teeth formation	• Acne or greasy skin
• Hair growth and colour	• Low fertility
• Energy production	• Pale skin
• Antioxidant in SOD	• Tendency to depression

Manganese

Sources

Tropical fruits, seeds, vegetables, berries

Functions	Signs linked with possible deficiency
• Component of bones, cartilage and tissues	• Muscle twitches
• Health of nervous system	• Childhood 'growing pains'
• Activates 20+ enzymes including SOD	• Dizziness or poor sense of balance
• Energy production	• Fits or convulsions
• Health of joints	• Sore knees
• Stabilizes blood sugar	
• Production of thyroxine	

Selenium

Sources

Seeds, seaweed – Molasses, mushrooms, cabbage, courgette
Seafood, liver, chicken

Functions	Signs linked with possible deficiency
• Antioxidant	• Family history of cancer
• Component of GP (Glutathione peroxidase) – anti-free radical	• Signs of premature aging
• Anti-inflammatory	• Cataracts
• Heart function	• High blood pressure
• Maintains eyes, hair and skin	• Frequent infections
• Essential for male reproductive capacity	
• Rolein thyroid function	

Chromium

Sources

Whole foods, whole grains, yeast, mushrooms, molasses
Oysters, eggs, chicken

Functions	Signs linked with possible deficiency
• Component of GTF (Glucose Tolerance Factor) role in blood sugar balance	• Excessive or cold sweats
• Normalizes appetite	• Dizziness or irritability after 6 hours without food
• Controls blood cholesterol	• Need for frequent meals
• Protects DNA and RNA	• Cold hands
• Essential for heart function	• Need for excessive sleep or drowsiness
• Stimulates production of nerve components	• Excessive thirst
	• Addicted to sweet foods

PROGRESS RECORD CHARTS

Positive Livetetics Elements ADDITIONS	Day 1	Day 2	Day 3	Day 4	Day 5	Day 6	Day 7	Week 3	Week 4
Daily Nourishment	Week 3 4	Week 3 4	Week 3 4	Week 3 4	Week 3 4	Week 3 4	Week 3 4		
Air/Breathing	5 x day								
Water	7 x day								
Fruit	5 x day								
Vegetables	5 x day								
Whole grains	3-5 x day								
Pulses/Beans	3-5 x day								
Nuts and seeds	1 x day								
Oil	1-2 x day								
Helpers									
Cranberry juice	2 x daily								
Cider vinegar	Daily								
Herbs and spices	Daily								
Supplementation									
Multinutrient	2 x day								
Antioxidant	1 x day								
Lifestyle									
Heart raising movement	Daily								
Stretching	Daily								
Resistance exercise	Daily								
Elimination									
Skin brush	Daily								
10-minute lie downs	2 x Daily								
Hot and cold shower	Daily								

Positive Livetetics Elements ADDITIONS	Day 1	Day 2	Day 3	Day 4	Day 5	Day 6	Day 7	Week 3	Week 4
Light & Air	Week 3 4	Week 3 4	Week 3 4	Week 3 4	Week 3 4	Week 3 4	Week 3 4		
Window open	Night								
30-minute outdoor walk	Daily								
Sleep									
8 hours' rest	Daily								
Relax									
Deliberate relaxation 20–30 mins	Daily								

Minimize or Eliminate SUBTRACTIONS	Day 1	Day 2	Day 3	Day 4	Day 5	Day 6	Day 7	Week 3	Week 4
D 'Foods'/Junk									
Sugar									
Tea, coffee and stimulants									
Colas/Sodas									
Alcohol									
Salt and salt snacks									
Chocolate and confectionery									
Artificial sweeteners									
Processed and 'ready' meals									
Take away									
Restaurant foods									
Wheat grains									
Dairy									
Meat									

Positive Livetetics Elements ADDITIONS		Day 1	Day 2	Day 3	Day 4	Day 5	Day 6	Day 7	Week 5	6
Daily Nourishment		Week 5 6	Week 5 6	Week 5 6	Week 5 6	Week 5 6	Week 5 6	Week 5 6		
Air/Breathing	5 x day									
Water	7 x day									
Fruit	5 x day									
Vegetables	5 x day									
Whole grains	3-5 x day									
Pulses/Beans	3-5 x day									
Nuts and seeds	1 x day									
Oil	1-2 x day									
Helpers										
Cranberry juice	2 x daily									
Cider vinegar	Daily									
Herbs and spices	Daily									
Supplementation										
Multinutrient	2 x day									
Antioxidant	1 x day									
Lifestyle										
Heart raising movement	Daily									
Stretching	Daily									
Resistance exercise	Daily									
Elimination										
Skin brush	Daily									
10-minute lie downs	2 x Daily									
Hot and cold shower	Daily									

Positive Livetetics Elements ADDITIONS		Day 1	Day 2	Day 3	Day 4	Day 5	Day 6	Day 7	Week 5	6
Light & Air		Week 5 6	Week 5 6	Week 5 6	Week 5 6	Week 5 6	Week 5 6	Week 5 6		
Window open	Night									
30-minute outdoor walk	Daily									
Sleep										
8 hours' rest	Daily									
Relax										
Deliberate relaxation 20–30 mins	Daily									

Minimize or Eliminate SUBTRACTIONS		Day 1	Day 2	Day 3	Day 4	Day 5	Day 6	Day 7	Week 5	6
D 'Foods'/Junk										
Sugar										
Tea, coffee and stimulants										
Colas/Sodas										
Alcohol										
Salt and salt snacks										
Chocolate and confectionery										
Artificial sweeteners										
Processed and 'ready' meals										
Take away										
Restaurant foods										
Wheat grains										
Dairy										
Meat										

Positive Livetetics Elements ADDITIONS		Day 1	Day 2	Day 3	Day 4	Day 5	Day 6	Day 7	Week 7	Week 8
Daily Nourishment		Week 7 8	Week 7 8	Week 7 8	Week 7 8	Week 7 8	Week 7 8	Week 7 8		
Air/Breathing	5 x day									
Water	7 x day									
Fruit	5 x day									
Vegetables	5 x day									
Whole grains	3-5 x day									
Pulses/Beans	3-5 x day									
Nuts and seeds	1 x day									
Oil	1-2 x day									
Helpers										
Cranberry juice	2 x daily									
Cider vinegar	Daily									
Herbs and spices	Daily									
Supplementation										
Multinutrient	2 x day									
Antioxidant	1 x day									
Lifestyle										
Heart raising movement	Daily									
Stretching	Daily									
Resistance exercise	Daily									
Elimination										
Skin brush	Daily									
10-minute lie downs	2 x Daily									
Hot and cold shower	Daily									

Positive Livetetics Elements ADDITIONS		Day 1	Day 2	Day 3	Day 4	Day 5	Day 6	Day 7	Week 7	8
Light & Air		Week 7 8	Week 7 8	Week 7 8	Week 7 8	Week 7 8	Week 7 8	Week 7 8		
Window open	Night									
30-minute outdoor walk	Daily									
Sleep										
8 hours' rest	Daily									
Relax										
Deliberate relaxation 20–30 mins	Daily									

Minimize or Eliminate SUBTRACTIONS	Day 1	Day 2	Day 3	Day 4	Day 5	Day 6	Day 7	Week 7	8
D 'Foods'/Junk									
Sugar									
Tea, coffee and stimulants									
Colas/Sodas									
Alcohol									
Salt and salt snacks									
Chocolate and confectionery									
Artificial sweeteners									
Processed and 'ready' meals									
Take away									
Restaurant foods									
Wheat grains									
Dairy									
Meat									

Positive Livetetics Elements ADDITIONS		Day 1	Day 2	Day 3	Day 4	Day 5	Day 6	Day 7	Week 9	10
Daily Nourishment		Week 9 10	Week 9 10	Week 9 10	Week 9 10	Week 9 10	Week 9 10	Week 9 10		
Air/Breathing	5 x day									
Water	7 x day									
Fruit	5 x day									
Vegetables	5 x day									
Whole grains	3-5 x day									
Pulses/Beans	3-5 x day									
Nuts and seeds	1 x day									
Oil	1-2 x day									
Helpers										
Cranberry juice	2 x daily									
Cider vinegar	Daily									
Herbs and spices	Daily									
Supplementation										
Multinutrient	2 x day									
Antioxidant	1 x day									
Lifestyle										
Heart raising movement	Daily									
Stretching	Daily									
Resistance exercise	Daily									
Elimination										
Skin brush	Daily									
10-minute lie downs	2 x Daily									
Hot and cold shower	Daily									

Positive Livetetics Elements ADDITIONS		Day 1	Day 2	Day 3	Day 4	Day 5	Day 6	Day 7	Week 9	10
Light & Air		Week 9 10	Week 9 10	Week 9 10	Week 9 10	Week 9 10	Week 9 10	Week 9 10		
Window open	Night									
30-minute outdoor walk	Daily									
Sleep										
8 hours' rest	Daily									
Relax										
Deliberate relaxation 20–30 mins	Daily									

Minimize or Eliminate SUBTRACTIONS	Day 1	Day 2	Day 3	Day 4	Day 5	Day 6	Day 7	Week 9	10
D 'Foods'/Junk									
Sugar									
Tea, coffee and stimulants									
Colas/Sodas									
Alcohol									
Salt and salt snacks									
Chocolate and confectionery									
Artificial sweeteners									
Processed and 'ready' meals									
Take away									
Restaurant foods									
Wheat grains									
Dairy									
Meat									

Positive Livetetics Elements ADDITIONS		Day 1	Day 2	Day 3	Day 4	Day 5	Day 6	Day 7	Week 1 1	1 2
Daily Nourishment		Week 11 12	Week 11 12	Week 11 12	Week 11 12	Week 11 12	Week 11 12	Week 11 12		
Air/Breathing	5 x day									
Water	7 x day									
Fruit	5 x day									
Vegetables	5 x day									
Whole grains	3-5 x day									
Pulses/Beans	3-5 x day									
Nuts and seeds	1 x day									
Oil	1-2 x day									
Helpers										
Cranberry juice	2 x daily									
Cider vinegar	Daily									
Herbs and spices	Daily									
Supplementation										
Multinutrient	2 x day									
Antioxidant	1 x day									
Lifestyle										
Heart raising movement	Daily									
Stretching	Daily									
Resistance exercise	Daily									
Elimination										
Skin brush	Daily									
10-minute lie downs	2 x Daily									
Hot and cold shower	Daily									

Positive Livetetics Elements ADDITIONS		Day 1	Day 2	Day 3	Day 4	Day 5	Day 6	Day 7	Week 11	12
Light & Air		Week 11 12	Week 11 12	Week 11 12	Week 11 12	Week 11 12	Week 11 12	Week 11 12		
Window open	Night									
30-minute outdoor walk	Daily									
Sleep										
8 hours' rest	Daily									
Relax										
Deliberate relaxation 20–30 mins	Daily									

Minimize or Eliminate SUBTRACTIONS	Day 1	Day 2	Day 3	Day 4	Day 5	Day 6	Day 7	Week 11	12
D 'Foods'/Junk									
Sugar									
Tea, coffee and stimulants									
Colas/Sodas									
Alcohol									
Salt and salt snacks									
Chocolate and confectionery									
Artificial sweeteners									
Processed and 'ready' meals									
Take away									
Restaurant foods									
Wheat grains									
Dairy									
Meat									

BIBLIOGRAPHY

Sources were taken from the following books:

Aihara, Herman, *Acid and Alkaline,* George Oshawa Macrobiotic Foundation, 1986

Holford, Patrick, *The Optimum Nutrition Bible,* Piatkus, 1999

Pottenger Jr. MD, Francis M, *Pottengers Cats,* Price Pottenger Nutrition Foundation, 1995

Bandler, Richard, *The Structure of Magic,* Science and Behaviour Books, 1975

Bandler, Richard, *Using your Brain,* Real People Press, 1985

Bandler, Richard and John Grinder, *Frogs into Princes,* Eden Grove, 1979

Barnard, Neal MD, *Food for Life,* Crown Publishers, 1993

Batmanghelidj, Dr F, *Your Body's Many Cries for Water,* Tagman, 2000

Bieler, Henry G MD, *Food is Your Best Medicine,* Ballantine, 1966

Cadbury, Deborah, *The Feminisation of Nature,* Hamish Hamilton, 1997

Cannon, Geoffrey, *Dieting Makes you Fat,* Century , 1983

Cannon, Geoffrey, *Superbug,* Virgin Books, 1995

Cannon, Geoffrey, *The Politics of Food,* Century Hutchinson, 1997

Carson, Rachel, *Silent Spring,* Houghton Miflin, 2002

Chaitow, Leon, *Principles of Fasting,* Thorsons, 1996

Cheraskin MD E, W M Ringsdorf Jr. MD and J W Clark DDS, *Diet and Disease,* Keats,1995

Cialdini, Robert B , *Influence - Science and Practice,* Allyn & Bacon, 2001

Clayton, Dr Paul, *Health Defence,* Accelerated Learning Systems, 2001

Cohen, *Milk the Deadly Poison,* Argus Publishing, 1998

Colborn, Theo, Dianne Dumanoski and John Peterson Myers, *Our Stolen Future,* Abacus, 1997

Coleman, Vernon, *Bodypower,* EMJ, 1999

Colgan, Dr Michael, *The New Nutrition,* Apple Publishing, 1995

Cooper MD, Kenneth, *Aerobics,* Bantam, 1968

Cousins, Norman, *Anatomy of an Illness,* Avon, 1992

Cox, Peter, *Why you don't need meat,* Thorsons, 1986

Cox, Peter and Peggy Bruseau, *Secret Ingredients,* Bantam, 1997

Crawford, Marsh, *Nutrition and Evolution,* Keats, 1995

Davies, Dr Stephen and Dr Alan Stewart, *Nutritional Medicine,* Pan, 1987

Dufty, William, *Sugar Blues,* Warner, 1975

Erasmus, Udo, *Fats that Heal, Fats that Kill,* Alive Books, 1986

Galland, Leo MD, *Four Pillars of Healing,* Random House, 1997

Gerson MD, Max, *A Cancer Therapy*, Gerson Institute, 1990

Hoffer MD, Abram, *Hoffers Laws of Natural Nutrition*, Quarry Press, 1996

Hoggan, Braly, *Dangerous Grains*, Avery, 2002

Holford, Patrick, *Optimum Nutrition for the Mind*, Piatkus, 2003

Hubbard, Bryan, *Secrets of the Drugs Industry*, WDDTY, 2002

Humphrys, John, *The Great Food Debate*, Hodder & Stoughton, 2001

Inlanader, Charles B, Lowell, S Levin and Ed Weiner, *Medicine on Trial*, Pantheon, 1988

Kenton, Leslie and Susannah , *Raw Energy*, Arrow, 1987

Kime MD MS, Zane R, *Sunlight*, World Health Publications, 1980

Klaper, Michael MD, *Pregnancy, Children and the Vegan Diet*, Gentle World, 1987

Lappe, Frances Moore, *Diet for a Samll Planet*, Ballantine, 1991

Lappe, Frances Moore and Joseph Collins, *Food First*, Ballantine, 1978

Lindlahr, Henry MD, *Natural Therapeutics* , CW Daniel, 1914

Lipski MS CCN, Elizabeth, *Digestive Wellness*, Keats, 1996

Mann, Charles C and Mark L Plummer, *The Aspirin Wars*, Harvard, 1991

Matsen MD, John , *Eating Alive*, Crompton, 1987

McCance and Widdowson, *The Composition of Foods* , RSC MAFF, 2000

McTaggart, Lynne, *What Doctors Don't Tell You*, Thorsons, 1996

Mendelsohn MD, Robert S, *Confessions of a Medical Heretic*, Contemporary Books, 1979

National Academy, *DRIs*, Institue of Medicine, 2000

Passwater PhD and A Richard, *Cancer Prevention and Nutritional Therapies*, Keats, 1983

Perretta, Lorraine, *Brain Food* , Hamlyn, 2001

Pilger, John, *Hidden Agendas*, Vintage, 1998

Price, Weston A DDS, *Nutrition and Physical Degeneration*, Price Pottenger, 1997

Rama Swami, Rudolph Ballentine M.D and Alan Hymes M.D., *Science of Breath*, Himalayan
    International Institute, 1979

Rifkin, Jeremy, *Beyond Beef*, Bantam, 1979

Robbins, John, *Diet for a New America*, Stillpoint, 1987

Robbins, John, *Diet for a New World*, Avon, 1992

Schlosser, Eric, *Fast Food Nation*, Allen Lane The Penguin Press, 2001

Sears PhD, Barry, *The Zone*, Harper Collins, 1995

Stauber, John and Sheldon Rampton, *Toxic Sludge is Good for You*, Common Courage, 1995

Tye, Larry, *The Father of Spin*, Owl Books, 1998

Walker, Martin, *Dirty Medicine*, Slingshot, 1993

Winter, Ruth MS, *Poisons in your Food*, Crown Publishers, 1991